CLEAN

10

CLEAN

The Revolutionary Program to Restore the Body's Natural Ability to Heal Itself

Alejandro Junger, M.D.

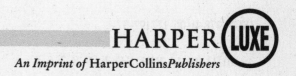

HARPER LUXE

An Imprint of HarperCollinsPublishers

FIRST HARPERLUXE EDITION

HarperLuxe™ is a trademark of HarperCollins Publishers.

Library of Congress Cataloging-in-Publication Data is available upon request.

ISBN 978-0-06-177497-3

10 11 12 13 RRD(H) 10 9 8 7 6 5

I dedicate this book to my daughter Grace,
my greatest teacher and doctor.
She provided the most profound experience of my
life, which is also the most powerful healing medicine:
unconditional love.

Contents

CHAPTER ONE

Why Clean?

Y ou are sitting on a familiar box, begging for pennies to survive, unaware that inside the box is a treasure that will not only fund this survival, but will also give you wealth beyond your wildest dreams.

You are not alone. Millions of Americans, like millions of others worldwide, are doing the same thing. Maybe you're begging for help to solve a small but troubling health problem, like extra weight, ongoing fatigue, allergies, depression, or a digestive disorder. Maybe you need help to avoid developing a bigger problem, like one of the so-called diseases of civilization—cardiovascular disease, cancer, obesity, and autoimmune disorders. Or maybe you want very much to look and feel younger and more radiant, and to slow down the onset of aging.

The pennies you are asking for are the prescription medications and surgeries that you have been taught are essential to remedy your problems. So you leave your hand out and collect what you can, waiting for the help promised to you by doctors, drug companies, and advertising.

But the truth is different. The power to heal lies somewhere much closer. You already have it, and you don't need prescriptions, treatments, or expensive experts to get it. In fact, you're sitting right on top of it.

That familiar box that's supporting you, almost unnoticed, is your own body, run by its incredible natural intelligence. The wealth beyond belief is the vibrant well-being and longevity that are your birthright.

And the treasure inside that will deliver this state of vitality, beauty, and vigor? It's something you probably haven't been taught to value. It's a system that is designed by nature to keep you healthy, youthful, and happy, if you only help it carry out its functions. It is the missing part of the health puzzle—an untapped source of healing, regeneration, restoration, and even rejuvenation. It is the on-board system that makes you and keeps you Clean, your system of detoxification.

This system, which comprises many organs and physiological processes working together throughout the body, is a wellspring of health. But its value has been forgotten. Modern medicine's fascination with molecules and micro-technology has targeted attention obsessively on smaller and smaller aspects of our biology while losing interest in looking at the big-picture systems in the body that keep us surviving and thriving. This is a mistake. Many of the health problems that trouble so many modern humans and cost society so much money can be alleviated when—instead of getting *more* detail-oriented in your approach, recruiting *more* superspecialists, inventing *more* technology, and adding in *more* medication—you take a broader perspective and do something simpler: turn your attention to the treasure that is already there, the detoxification system, and reactivate its potential.

A focused period of detoxifying is a reset for the whole physical and mental body. It delivers an all-access pass to boundless reserves of energy you didn't know you had. You find that every part of your body works better, imbalances are rectified, and irritating symptoms get a chance to melt away on their own—all by your simply "switching on" a system that you were born with and that has been patiently waiting to serve you.

Imagine your right arm has been taped to the side of your body since birth. You grow up using only your left arm, thinking this is normal, because everyone else was exactly the same. As an adult you take on carpentry, and your business starts doubling each year. Just when you are about to collapse from the intense work-load, a stranger rings your doorbell. He untapes your right arm, and to your surprise, without ever having dreamed of it as a possibility, you accelerate from a state of overload, unable to fulfill your orders, to op-erating up to your unbounded true potential and doing more than ever before.

The stranger arriving at the door is the Clean pro-gram contained in this book. Untaping that arm is the act of uncovering and accelerating the detoxification system's full potential. The flourishing productivity that results is your body's natural ability to maintain steady energy, avoid colds and the flu, heal allergies, age grace-fully, and avoid disease.

Who is a candidate for using this program? Every-one who lives a modern life, eats a modern diet, and inhabits the modern world.

For thousands of years, humanity has recognized the existence of toxic influences that cause dysfunction, damage, disease, premature aging, and death. These toxins have the potential to irritate and stress us and ul-timately cause the body to suffer in many ways, small and large, from the unmeasurable realm of thought and emotion to the material chemicals generated as the waste by-products of our cells' daily life. Ancient cultures also knew that we are equipped with a grand system of detoxification, which is the result of the harmonious collaboration of several smaller systems. This system is continuously working; in fact, it keeps us alive every second of every minute of every day. If the body didn't constantly coordinate its complex symphony of activities, these waste products would build up, we would become sick, and we would eventually die. The "baseline" detox mode that is occurring at every moment of our lives is part of the basic formula of life. It makes our very existence possible.

What the older traditions of healing understood very well was the crucial importance of harnessing the detoxification system and using it to our advantage in order to achieve our maximum mental, emotional, and physical potential. The sages and healers of many cultures, across borders and eras, all possessed the knowledge that this grand system must periodically be allowed to enter a deeper detox mode than its ordinary day-to-day function in order to handle the accumulation of toxins that can build up so easily in times of excess eating, activity, and stress.

Practitioners of these early healing traditions understood that resting some of the major body systems, especially the digestive system, was integral to life. Fasting, silent retreats, and contemplative times were considered essential to a peaceful, healthy, and fulfilling experience of life. It wasn't just an esoteric concept. Human beings' genetic evolution—the way our bodies work best—has been shaped by the fasting that was imposed on us by the hunter-gatherer way of life. For millennia, humans experienced periods of *feasting* followed by periods of imposed famine. Long periods of having an empty belly were inescapable, but this proved to be a key to health. The detoxification system could switch on and stay on with plenty of time and energy to do its essential cleanup work, liberating the body of a whole backload of waste products trapped inside, because it wasn't competing with the digestive system for fuel.

Today, life has changed. We are newly waking up to something of an evolutionary paradox. The more the toxicity of modern life increases, bombarding us with unnatural toxins from our diet and the environment, the more the demands to *detoxify* have increased. Yet our body's ability to handle the load hasn't accelerated at the same rapid pace. How could it? The world might have changed dramatically in one century, but our bodies take many generations to make one genetic change. The more dangerously toxic life has become, and the more depleted of vital nutrients our diets have become, and the more rushed life has become, the more our grand detoxification system has gotten overwhelmed. It is almost hibernating: it is still there, doing the daily "baseline" work that allows us to live, but it is faltering under the additional twenty-first-century burden of poor diet, environmental toxins, and stress.

We are all dealing with the effects of this to different degrees. Commonplace complaints such as headaches, bowel irregularities, allergies, weight problems, depression, anxiety, and pain are largely caused by failing detox systems. Looking older, feeling more tired, and losing the radiant luster of health are also directly related to this overburdened state. Yet all of this can be reversed and, frequently, healed when we pay attention to detoxification.

Tragically, most premature deaths today are a direct result of failing detox systems. One of the most common consequences of poor detoxification functioning is inflammation, the body's necessary, but now dangerously overused, survival strategy. Modern medicine has only recently awakened to the fact that chronic inflammation is a common condition underlying the diseases that have become epidemics today, including cancer, cardiovascular disease, diabetes, and autoimmune disorders. Yet it is still blind to the root of the problem, the toxicity of modern life, and our bodies' weakness in dealing with it. Only when we start the treatment there, targeting the seed of the problem, can we truly begin to ward off disease.

When I first consulted with Ellen at the Eleven Eleven Wellness Center in downtown Manhattan where I see patients several days a week, she was frustrated. After her yearly physical exam her doctor had told her she needed to take medication to lower her blood pressure. She was extremely reluctant to do so, because she believed there had to be a more natural way to lower it, but her physician offered no alternative, instead presenting her with what she described as a "case closed, God has spoken" diagnosis and a prescribed course of drug treatment. It didn't suit her; she was someone who wanted a partner in building her own health, not a dependency on expensive medication. She also sensed that taking chemical drugs daily would have a taxing effect on her body, though she couldn't explain exactly why.

To start her on the path to lowering her blood pressure, I asked Ellen to do the Clean program. She hesitated for just a moment, concerned that it would disrupt her performance at work too much, but told me she was so eager to avoid blood pressure medications that some inconvenience didn't matter to her. She followed the program to the letter, maintaining her usual five-day-a-week exercise routine but toning down its intensity slightly. After completing Clean, Ellen's results were impressive: her blood pressure decreased by 25 percent, she lost 21 pounds, her body-fat percentage dropped by 7 percent and her cholesterol levels fell by 40 percent. She was never hungry, had plenty of energy, and slept soundly. Even her physician congratulated her on her results. By putting some of her regular eating habits on hold and resting her digestive system, Ellen had initiated a way for her body to find its way back to health. By taking early action, she had lowered the high blood pressure and high cholesterol that, untreated, could have landed her in a cardiologist's office.

Detoxification has become a primary area of concern; I created the Clean program to boost this essential function, and it is a tool I use frequently in my practice. Although as a physician I specialize in diseases of the heart, I am constantly amazed by the ability of a detoxification program to transform all aspects of my patients' well-being in such a simple, commonsense manner. Many of those trained in Western medicine still view "cleansing" as an activity done on the fringes of alternative healing. But the integrative model of medicine combines the wisdom of old and new, and today my understanding of detoxification is in complete resonance with what I learned during years of medical school training and practice. Detoxification as a complete and essential wellspring of health was never presented to us Western-trained doctors in the complete way that I understand it today, yet its power to heal was always there, right under our noses.

This book and the cleansing-detoxifying program it presents have grown out of the experience of helping many people jump-start their way back to the higher levels of health they deserve—becoming slimmer, brighter, happier, more resilient, and less burdened by poor health conditions that once slowed down their lives. It will clearly distinguish for you the connection between toxicity and most diseases. In fact, I think "disease" should be written "dis-ease," to highlight the loss of a sense of well-being and ease, in addition to outright illness, that result from toxicity. *Clean* will show you how toxins, far from being invisible agents floating somewhere "out there" in the environment, actually enter your body and corrode it from the inside. As toxicity accumulates, your body systems are damaged one by one, starting with your intestines.

You will discover how the early signs and symptoms of toxicity are confused and ignored in our culture, often written off as the "normal" wear and tear on our body parts, as if nothing can be done. This failure to catch the early symptoms means that more serious signs and symptoms appear later on. Typically they are suppressed by means of drugs and surgery, and once more the underlying primary cause remains unexamined and unaddressed. Finally, overburdened with toxicity, one or more systems in the body collapse and the chronic diseases that take so much effort to manage and mediate set in.

Modern medicine is still blind to this toxicity-disease connection. Instead, doctors generally wait until a "crash" happens in the form of an acute, emergency problem, and then they desperately call in the big guns (harsh drugs and surgery) to save the day. This medical artillery only adds to the toxic burden; instead of healing the problem at the root, the treatment results in more toxic residue for the body to eliminate.

Clean will reveal to you the connections that—like that familiar box you didn't think to open but have been sitting on for years—have been ignored by most of society and most of modern medicine. It explains how intestinal irritation caused by dietary and environmental toxicity can present as a range of symptoms you might never have thought could be connected to toxicity, such as seasonal allergies, skin rashes, depression, or simply a lack of enthusiasm for life. *Clean* provides clarity among the hundreds of different cleansing-detox programs that have flooded our market and explains the science that ties them all together. It details what these toxins are, where they are, how you are exposed to them, and how they affect your life and health. It is a primer to surviving and thriving in a toxic world.

But more important, *Clean* will give you the tools to reactivate your detoxification system to its fullest, giving it a chance to go into deep-cleaning mode and restore your body's own ability to heal, regenerate, and even rejuvenate itself. The Clean program is a simple, safe, and medically proven way to put this powerful ancient knowledge to work in practical, modern ways. It will show you how a cleansing-detox program does not have to be disruptive to daily life or make you feel deprived. It can be incorporated into a regular schedule and support your need for energy while gradually eliminating the toxins that have blocked optimal functioning of body and mind. You can start slowly on your first-ever cleanse by doing a one-week program, make a bigger commitment with a fourteen-day program, or jump right in for a full commitment of three weeks. Whether you complete seven, fourteen, or twenty-one days of Clean, every day spent on the program will help you avoid becoming one of the statistics that we hear of constantly, telling you that heart disease, cancer, and other modern diseases are almost inevitable and that with aging comes degeneration, hospitalization, and dependency. Each time you Clean, you are empowering your own ability to create, and then sustain, the high level of health that your body is so well equipped to experience.

WHAT IS CLEAN?

Clean is a tool that anybody can use for restoring, rebalancing, and healing. Designed with the needs of busy people in mind, Clean is a simple and practical detoxification plan that fits into day-to-day life instead of asking you to put your life on hold. It is different from other detox plans that are gaining popularity in beauty and alternative-health circles, such as intensive juicing or fasting plans or the milder raw-foods diets. Extensive clinical and personal experience has shown me that these practices demand too much time, energy, or attention for most people. They work best for those who have already done months or years of dietary cleanup, and they are better suited to retreat settings. Such demanding programs can even in some cases be dangerous. Stripping away waste materials from the body without simultaneously carefully replenishing essential nutrients can cause a state in which toxicity is increased, not reduced. Intensive detox programs can leave a person depleted or, worse, in danger.

Clean is designed with safety and effectiveness in mind. It is backed by cutting-edge scientific understanding of how our organs, hormones, and enzymes function. At its core, however, are these very simple easy-to-understand concepts:

1. Toxins and stress create obstacles for the normal functioning and self-healing capabilities of our bodies.
2. Modern eating habits and lifestyles pollute our bodies and don't provide the nutrients necessary for them to function at optimum levels.
3. By removing the obstacles and providing what is lacking, our bodies bounce back into health, energy is restored, and we begin to look and feel our best.

The Clean program breaks down into three one-week plans, with a preliminary phase consisting of an elimination diet to prepare for the cleanse. Ultimately, you will work your way toward a three-week cleanse. It will be your choice whether to take Clean all the way through and complete the three-week program, or to work up to the three-week cleanse in incremental phases, completing a slightly longer program each time you do it (in most cases I recommend doing Clean once a year). Know that any step taken in the Clean direction will have positive impact, and over the long term doing cleanses on a regular basis will have a cumulative effect.

THREE STEPS OF CLEAN

One-Week Cleanse. Your first three to five days on the program will be a lesson in how the body resists changing the deeply engrained habits around eating and drinking, even habits that your mind understands to be toxic and wants to let go of. You are encouraged to finish at least the first full week of Clean; by the end of this time you will experience a surge of vibrant energy and clarity of mind, as toxins are released from the tissues they have been trapped in and are recirculated for neutralization and subsequent elimination.

One week is enough time for your body to take advantage of this new state that you are creating. The Clean program optimizes the conditions needed for our bodies to fully express their miraculous potential of regeneration, repair, and healing. You will also have an opportunity to explore one of the dysfunctions that keeps Americans overweight: hunger. We so commonly say "I'm hungry," but most of us don't really know what hunger is. That bodily sensation that you call hunger may be something different. During Clean, you will finally be able to rename that sensation for what it really is. Clean guides you through a very effective way of doing just that.

More important, it is very likely that by the time you complete your first week, your motivation will soar and you'll continue on. Some of my successful cases started with patients who were skeptics and gave me just a few days to prove my theory to them in practice.

Two-Week Cleanse. If you are able to continue, don't stop. Set a goal of carrying straight on and accomplishing a second week on the program. Two weeks on Clean will deliver to you greater benefits, as systems in your body that had been blocked and slowed begin to be optimized again, while other systems that had been on "red alert" to help you survive the insult of the toxic world get soothed and settled. Long-standing symptoms of imbalance on the "surface," such as skin problems, weight issues, allergies, and intestinal issues, begin to disappear.

Three-Week Cleanse. The completion of your third week will show you how it feels to slow down and even reverse the aging process. You are able to feel how vital, clear, and optimistic you should really feel for your true physical age, not your chronological age. The transformation in those who follow the Clean program in its entirety is often remarkable. They finally drop stubborn pounds. Their complexions firm, tighten, and glow. The whites of the eyes get whiter and brighter. They sleep more soundly and have a higher energy level throughout the day. Patients can finally find relief from many of the discomforts that they have been struggling to get rid of, from constipation to sinus infections to joint pain. Disease processes assumed to be chronic or only manageable by drugs are often slowed down and even reversed. As you experience your body's ability to restore order on its own, you will no longer see conditions that once had a frightening hold on you, from high blood pressure to high cholesterol and more, as life sentences.

Improved physiological balance can have a positive effect on psychological and emotional levels too. Moods improve, and a sense of mental clarity returns. After completing the program, many find that their cravings are reduced, poor foods and highly caffeinated drinks lose their appeal, and a mindful relationship to meals is restored. Most report that their work and relationships get a boost from what they can only describe as a heightened state of self-awareness. At a level beyond the physical, completing the three-step Clean program can feel like cleaning dirty spectacles: you get a fresh vision of your world.

THE IMPORTANCE OF A WELLNESS PLAN

A plan is essential to any endeavor where we want to see growth and success. We make a business plan, investing time and money, on a new startup. We spend huge amounts of time and money hiring experts to help us make savings plans, wedding plans, career plans, vacation plans—and sometimes even funeral plans. What this comes down to is breaking a big task into small, achievable steps and putting them on a calendar. Such planning makes a goal much easier to achieve. Yet in many years of working in medicine, I have rarely met a patient with a Wellness Plan.

As you'll learn in chapter 8, in order to truly survive in a toxic world, you need to put a Wellness Plan in place. A reasonable yet organized Wellness Plan that sets out small goals for the year empowers you to achieve the ongoing state of health you need to thrive in our toxic world. Conventional health-care protocols do not cover all the bases that are essential for ongoing health in our stressed environment. For example, almost no family doctors routinely test for vitamin D levels, something I believe should be a priority, nor do they help you decide which supplements to take and when. Should you want to test for certain lingering toxins, you're also usually on your own. I'll show you how this, too, can be achieved on your plan for the year.

The Clean detox program helps you get clarity on your health goals and priorities. It can also be used to bring you back on track when your commitment to good eating weakens and you deviate for a few weeks. Like a mile marker you can always find your way back to, Clean can realign you with your Wellness Plan and get you back on track.

Clean is safe for almost everyone. Note, however, that all cleanses can have an effect on the way prescription medications are absorbed. Some treatment regimens will exclude you as a candidate for a detox program. If you are currently taking prescription medications, please read on carefully before proceeding with the program.

THE CLEAN AUDIT

Answer the questions on this list and note your "yes" answers.

Do you have headaches more than occasionally?
Do you tend to get colds or viruses each year?
Do you have bowel movements less frequently
    than after every meal?

Do you have bowel movements that are not soft
and easily passed?

Do you have diarrhea more than very rarely?

Do you get itchy or watery eyes and nose at certain
times of year?

Do you have allergies or hay fever?

Do you often get congested or mucusy?

Do you get bloated after eating?

Do you have extra pounds that won't come off
with diet and exercise?

Do you have puffiness in areas of your face or
body?

Do you have dark circles under your eyes?

Do you get heartburn?

Do you have gas more than occasionally?

Do you have bad breath or body odor?

Is there a thin white coat on the back of your
tongue when you wake up?

Do you get cravings for certain kinds of food,
especially sugary, starchy, or dairy foods?

Do you have a tendency toward restless sleep?

Do you have itchy skin, pimples, or any other
troubling skin condition?

Do you get pain or stiffness in your joints or
muscles?

Do you have low moods or a foggy mind?

Do you find that you are forgetful, have difficulty concentrating, or can't find words?

Do you feel apathetic and tired?

Do you feel anger or bursts of irrational frustration?

Do you have higher than average sensitivity to odors?

Have you noticed an increasing sensitivity to toxins in everyday life, such as feeling more nauseated when you smell dry-cleaning fluid or fill up your car's tank with gas, noticing stronger effects of certain food additives, or having reactions to cleaning or personal-care products?

Do you use multiple prescription medications?

Do you use many potentially toxic chemicals in your home or work environment?

Do you have musculoskeletal aches and pains or symptoms suggestive of fibromyalgia?

Do you have tingling or numbness on one side?

Do you have strange reactions to medications or supplements?

Do you have recurrent edema?

Have you noticed a worsening of any troublesome symptoms after anesthesia or pregnancy?

These could all be symptoms of toxicity. It's hard to find anyone who doesn't answer "yes" to at least one or two of these questions. Some people have many more "yes" answers than that. Whatever your response, affirmative answers to any of these questions indicate that you would benefit highly from Clean, which has been shown to improve and clear up these symptoms and many others.

Clean is not a magic bullet. It is not designed to cure every ailment. It is designed to be a jump start—a reboot that gets all systems running better. Once you've completed part or all of it the first time, it is a preventive tool that you'll use periodically to shed accumulated toxins and switch on deeper healing. Meanwhile, you will create an ongoing Wellness Plan to achieve a set of longer-term toxin-beating goals.

Clean is not the result of multimillion-dollar clinical trials or pharmaceutical company sponsorship. This modern detox program came to life in the same way that many great discoveries are made, when one person went on a journey to find a solution for his own suffering. In the case of Clean, that person was me.

CHAPTER TWO

A Doctor's Journey

I was born in Uruguay in 1964 to Jewish parents who survived World War II. My mother left Germany days after she was born. My father survived a concentration camp in Hungary and went to Uruguay after the war, looking for his sisters. He found them, and my mom.

Life in Montevideo and Punta del Este was slow-paced. We shopped at the local farmers' market and almost always had lunch or dinner sitting at the dining-room table, all together as a family. Our city was safe, and children played in the streets without supervision.

Early on I knew what I wanted to do when I grew up: I wanted to become a doctor and help alleviate people's suffering; help them become healthier and live longer and better lives. I went to medical school and fell in love with medicine. Our family doctors used to do house visits, spend hours with us, and teach us all kinds of interesting things. I wanted to be like them.

When I graduated, I decided to become a cardiologist. Something about the heart attracted my interest. The fast thinking necessary, the life-saving decisions made in a split second, the satisfaction of saving someone's life without having to wait for months to see if the pills were going to work—all these things left me with no doubt of my choice of specialty.

After graduating I wanted to study in the place where my medical school textbooks had been written. I got a position as an intern at New York University's Downtown Hospital in Lower Manhattan and moved there a week after my graduation to complete three years of training in Internal Medicine. At the end of the three years I was twenty-six years old.

Life in Manhattan moved at a lightning-fast pace, very different from my home. Medical training was tough. Being on call for up to three days in a row, always busy, I had no time to prepare meals. My main sources of nourishment were takeout, vending machines, nurses' potlucks (lots of them), and the hospital cafeteria. If I had some extra time, I visited the nearest supermarket. I was fascinated by all the packages, the colors, the smells, and the fact that with a microwave oven, anyone could have a dinner in minutes. I felt like an aboriginal who finds himself in the magical modern city, and I often found myself thinking, "Boy, these Americans really know how to make things easy."

But life as a trainee doctor in one of the busiest cities in the world started taking a toll on me. I was gaining weight and started sneezing like crazy with every change of season. I was exhausted, but could not get much sleep. Overall I still enjoyed the experience of learning from doctors, some of whom were considered the top in their field. As to the deterioration in my well-being, I figured, "Once I graduate, things will change."

After three years of internship and residency, I moved to Manhattan's Upper East Side and started my training in cardiology at Lenox Hill Hospital. Running the Cardiac Intensive Care Unit, admitting patients from the emergency room, and consulting all over the hospital added the weight of responsibility to my shoulders and the weight of bagels to my belly. In those second three years of training my allergies got so bad that I had to take antihistamines and use steroid inhalers several times. My digestion was turning into a nightmare. I was often bloated, and I had abdominal discomfort and alternating bouts of constipation and diarrhea. This was alarming.

I decided to ask one of our attending gastroenterologists for help. Within minutes of listening to my story, he ordered an upper and a lower endoscopy, abdominal sonogram, and full blood work. Every test came back absolutely normal. The specialist's diagnosis was "irritable bowel syndrome." Not much could be done, I was told, except try to control symptoms with antispasmodics, antiflatulence pills, painkillers, and antidiarrhea medication alternating with laxatives. Nobody asked me what I was eating—which was not surprising, since I had never had a nutrition class myself.

A few months before finishing my fellowship I started waking up with chest pain. If I hadn't already been a cardiologist myself by then, I would have gone to see one, but I knew the heart muscle and its arteries were not the problem. That other aspect of the heart, the one I had not had a single class or discussion about in all my years of training, was the problem. I was sad. In fact, I was depressed.

This to me was unbelievable. There was no history of depression in my family. My life was busy, but I liked working hard and I was good at what I did. Something was very wrong, because my feeling of impending doom was not justified by whatever difficulties I had at that time.

And soon I started noticing something even more alarming: from the moment I woke up until the moment I went to bed, my mind did not stop thinking.

There were always thoughts rolling through my mind. It was not me choosing to think them. In fact, if I had a choice I wouldn't be thinking 90 percent of the thoughts that were happening day in and out. Sometimes there were dialogues in my mind. I noticed that there was only one difference between crazy people talking to themselves in the subway and me: they were doing it out loud.

The thoughts were louder at night. I could not sleep. Which only led to more thoughts. If *I* was not choosing those thoughts, who was? Where were they coming from? Was I going mad?

At one point it got so bad that I decided to seek help from a top psychiatrist in New York. After one session of questions he solemnly said, "You are depressed. You have a chemical imbalance." He explained that my brain was not producing enough serotonin. He wrote me a prescription for Prozac. In the elevator on my way out of his office building I looked at the piece of paper in my hand and wondered, "How did my cells forget to do their chemistry? How did they become imbalanced?"

I didn't like the idea of taking a medication for the rest of my life, so I decided to get a second opinion. It took the new psychiatrist two sessions before he declared, "You have a chemical imbalance in your brain," and wrote a prescription for Zoloft, a cousin of Prozac. This doctor talked a little longer, saying that a chemical called serotonin, a neurotransmitter, is responsible for the feeling of well-being, of happiness. He said my serotonin was low. Zoloft would ultimately raise the levels of serotonin in my brain and resolve my symptoms. When I asked him what had *caused* my cells to reduce the production of serotonin, he answered that it was not well understood, but that I was not alone. He was starting to see depression in almost epidemic proportions.

Instinctively I rejected the idea of being on prescription drugs for the rest of my life. The psychiatrists had no answers to my questions. Neither did a number of other therapists, social workers, teachers, and friends whom I asked. I wondered if anyone else would be able to satisfy my need to understand what was happening. So I started going to bookstores. I quickly discovered that New York has amazing bookstores (even more impressive than its supermarkets) where a person could sit and study for hours without buying a thing. I took full advantage, starting my research in the psychiatry and psychology shelves. "Thinking" . . . "thought" . . . "the mind" . . . I read everything I could get my hands on to answer my burning questions: Where are my thoughts coming from? How are they affecting my feelings to the point of despair? How can I stop this madness?

Every time I read something that resonated with me, I made a note of the reference, and immediately I'd go look up the book that was referenced. In this way I found myself shifting from the psychiatry section into the self-help section and then into the New Age section of the bookstore.

One day, following the trail of references, I found myself looking for a book in the Eastern Philosophy section. As I was browsing the shelves, a book literally "fell" on my hands and opened up to a chapter titled "Meditation: Silencing the Mind." As I read the first few paragraphs, it was as if the skies were opening up. It said that through the practice of meditation one could slow down and even stop the incessant habitual thinking process. The mind was described as the "monkey mind," always moving from one thing to another, always busy; some people also call it "radio playing." This information was exactly what I was looking for.

I laughed at how close the names of these two approaches were: medication and meditation. So close and yet so far apart. I immediately made up my "monkey mind." I had to meditate.

Finding a meditation teacher was not easy. After a couple of awkward experiences, my friend Fernando offered to take me to a specialist. We drove upstate to a school of meditation that same day. It's a monastery of sorts, where seekers can come to study and learn. This meditation school was led by an Indian meditation master. As soon as I met her there was no doubt in my mind she would have some of the answers to my questions. She was fully present to such degree and so profoundly calm within that it was felt by everyone around her. I had such an intense experience from simply being in her presence that my thinking brain fell completely silent for some time. When my mind started the incessant radio playing again, it was different: I could remember the experience of silence. I had a reference point. I had a sneak preview of what was possible—and I resolved to acquire that ability, to silence my mind, to become present. The course of my life changed at that moment, and it has never been the same.

I started reading all the books that this Indian teacher had written, and the ones her teacher had written before. I also drove every weekend to the meditation courses offered at the school of meditation at that time. On one of these weekends, an announcement was made that a volunteer doctor was needed for the medical clinic at their meditation school in India. A series of magical synchronicities ended with a firm decision: I would go to India. To the shock of my colleagues and family I turned down all the offers I'd had to join very lucrative cardiology practices, packed my bags, and left.

In India I studied yoga. I learned how the physical movement routines that were starting to be a great fashion in America were only one aspect of yoga. There are eight "limbs" of yoga in total: *yamas*, personal attitudes toward the world and others; *niyamas*, attitudes toward self; *asanas*, body postures; *pranayama*, breathing exercises; *pratyahara*, control of the senses; *dharana*, concentration; *dhyana*, meditation; and *samadhi*, enlightenment, firmness in the present moment. It is an expansion of awareness and opening of the mind. And that was exactly what happened to me.

As my form of service I directed a team of volunteer health practitioners from all over the world. There were Ayurvedic doctors, Chinese medicine doctors, chiropractors, nurses, massage therapists, hands-on healers, meditation instructors, and many other practitioners, all with different philosophies and all practicing different techniques. Our mission was to treat the meditation school's large population of students and to take our traveling hospital—a converted school bus— to the surrounding villages, some of the poorest places on the planet. We took on every case as a team, discussing each patient's condition from everyone's point of view. It was a truly integrative approach. I had never heard of "integrative medicine" before, but suddenly I was practicing it.

As I heard the other doctors explain their views on patients and diseases, I was blown away by how much sense they made. Even more impressive were the results I was witnessing from using herbs, acupuncture, diet, massage, chiropractic care, and hands-on healing. These were being used in a subtler way than Western medicine knew—to find the root cause of imbalance in the body and mind, not just put out the fires of symptoms. It struck me that what we were practicing could not be categorized as "alternative" or "traditional." It was, simply, common sense. On certain occasions a Western medical approach using drugs or surgery was absolutely necessary, and the advanced technology available was life-saving. But this was rarely needed. Given the right support and conditions, the body's natural healing ability was restored without drug intervention. My mind, which had been rigorously schooled in the paradigm of conventional medicine, was cracked wide open. And meanwhile, my own mental and physical health, though far from optimal, were getting better by the week.

By the end of my year of volunteering at the meditation school I had erased many categories of medicine from my mind: "alternative," "traditional," "Western," "allopathic," "Eastern," "Ayurvedic," "Chinese." All these medical traditions and practices blended into one integrative category that I called "open-minded medicine." It was, I decided, the process of bringing the best of Eastern and Western medicines to the table without judgment in order to best serve each and every patient as a unique individual. By the time I returned to the United States, I was determined to bring this new style of practicing medicine into the hospital system—to change it from within. I returned to the States and took a job as an attending cardiologist in a busy practice in Palm Springs, California, with admitting privileges in the four local hospitals.

Before I knew it I was back in the all-American rat race—personally and professionally. It was much harder to maintain peace and well-being here than it had been at the meditation school. Constant commuting in the car, responding to beepers, and inserting pacemakers and IV drips became my reality. The pressure was on to make the rounds of wards and intensive-care units as fast as possible, to keep the practice profitable. On paper the job was enviable. If I stuck it out, in three years I'd be a partner in a very successful practice. But treating patients this way was killing my spirit. I had no time to listen to my patients' symptoms or even recognize their basic humanity. They received, on average, seven minutes of attention, and the system treated them like commodities: a way to do more tests, write more prescriptions, and make more money. The patients who came to me were often taking five or more prescription drugs. Neither I nor they completely understood how all these chemicals interacted in their bodies. The system was set up to encourage someone in my position to add more medications to the already full load. This was not the dream of healing I'd grown up with.

Not surprisingly, the effects of stress, cafeteria food, and late-night dinners piled up again. My own symptoms of irritable bowel syndrome (IBS) and the foggy mental state that before had made me sad now returned. In private moments I had to ask myself if my health was much better than my patients'.

Things changed abruptly again one day with the arrival of an unannounced visitor. My friend Eric, a stressed-out movie producer, showed up at my Palm Springs house. I almost fainted when I saw him. Ten days before he'd been his usual bloated, overweight, sallow-skinned self. Now a different man stood before me: fifteen pounds lighter, with shiny glowing skin, and with eyes whose whites were whiter than any I'd ever seen. He was also exuding a sense of calm and joy that were highly out of character. Sensing my astonishment, he told me he'd just completed a detox program at a holistic center located minutes from my home, out in the desert. He'd abandoned his usual routine of restaurant meals, alcohol, and all-night movie shoots for a retreat based on green juices, colonics, massage, sunshine, yoga, and meditation. This shiny new being was the result.

It was an "Aha!" moment for me. This was exactly the kind of result I wanted to offer to my patients. I got the address of the center, named the We Care spa, and signed up for my own program.

With my overloaded schedule, I had to improvise. Instead of booking myself in as a guest, I drove to the center on my lunch breaks, where I would fill my jars with fresh juices and take natural supplements. Every day I'd get a colonic hydrotherapy treatment to help flush out the toxins that were getting released from my tissues via my intestines. And then I'd go back to work until late at the multiple busy offices under my care. I committed to two weeks of this intensive juice fasting program and made sure to keep my mind wide open, because although I'd trained hard in fitness in the past and had months of eating very simply and wholesomely in India, this was different from anything I'd ever done.

By the third day of the detox program, my fatigue, hunger, and headaches had disappeared. By the seventh day, my IBS had completely vanished and has so far only threatened to return at times when I disregarded my lessons. After two weeks of following the center's cleansing program, my depression—or whatever was left of it—had completely lifted and I had lost fifteen pounds, just like my friend. I had not felt better since my teens.

I was floored. My own body had reset itself. The irritation I'd been experiencing in different areas—mood, energy levels, allergies, and digestive function—had all been connected. They were different ways that my body was showing it was toxic, damaged, and out of balance. By detoxing, I had restored that balance and repaired the damage. As a result, my cells were remembering how to do their chemistry. My guts were restored their normal functioning without medication, and my serotonin levels had gone up. Nobody I'd consulted in modern medicine had suggested these separate symptoms were linked—or had told me that I could heal them myself. It was knowledge that no medical school or specialist seemed to possess. Several times a day, colleagues stopped me at the hospital and said, "Alex, you look ten years younger!" I wondered, had I just reversed the aging process? Was that even possible? If so, it was a subject that—just like nutrition—was missing from my medical school curriculum.

This was a turning point. I finally saw my path clearly. I quit my job at the hospitals and moved to Los Angeles, one of the most polluted cities in the world but also, luckily, home to some of the most progressive thinkers and health practitioners in the world—and lots of open-minded patients. I started studying everything I could about detoxification, from the ancient traditions to the new scientific studies that had come out explaining the biochemistry of detoxification in detail. I immersed myself in the study of the emerging field of Functional Medicine, which translates the Eastern paradigm of health to fit the Western terminology and tools with incredibly effective results. Every week I drove back to the desert for two days and worked as the medical consultant for the We Care spa. Susana Belen, the center's visionary founder and owner, and I guided many different kinds of people through their juice fasting experiences, developing our understanding of the process and sharing our findings with each other and the guests.

I began to treat patients as an M.D. and cardiologist who worked with an expanded toolkit. It still contained lab tests, medications, and surgical interventions when needed. It also contained detoxing, aspects of Chinese medicine, and a huge emphasis on dietary change to build wellness from the inside. It was my vision of open-minded medicine, and I had finally come full circle—putting the pieces of my own story into practice with others.

In those early days, I sent many of my Los Angeles patients to We Care and watched them have similar transformations through detoxing, sometimes coming back to life after long periods of dealing with uncomfortable symptoms. But leaving town wasn't practical or affordable for everyone, so I started to research and design a way to achieve the same results without the need to go on retreat, a way of detoxing that everyone could afford. This is what I present to my patients and to you as the Clean program.

CHAPTER THREE

Global Toxicity: Another Inconvenient Truth

E ver since my first consultation with a psychiatrist in New York, I constantly found myself asking, "How and why did my brain cells forget their chemistry?"

The low serotonin level in my brain, which I was told explained the problem, was simply a description of *what* happens when the chemistry is forgotten by the neurons. I wanted to find out *how* and *why*. In medicine, understanding how and why is the real "diagnosis." This is what doctors do.

Doctors used to pride themselves on diagnosing a problem by observation and deduction: they'd take a good patient history, listen, and observe. Modern doctors, pressed for time and fearful of lawsuits, heavily rely on blood tests, X-rays, sonograms, endoscopy, and many other laboratory evaluations. In India, working out of our bus–turned–mobile-hospital, with no equipment other than a stethoscope, our ears, eyes, and noses, my colleagues and I returned to the simpler methods of observation. Eastern schools of medicine don't see patients as isolated from their environment— including family, village, and spiritual path. Changes in environment or the predominant quality of one's thoughts are considered equally important as changes in body temperature. All aspects of a patient's life are believed to affect each other significantly and play a role in the maintenance of well-being. The root of disease is also found this way, by looking at both the bigger and the smaller picture together. Physical, mental, emotional, social, and environmental symptoms are all taken into consideration when making a diagnosis. Finding the common thread that ties them together often reveals the underlying imbalance at the origin of disease.

Back in the United States, chronic diseases were on the rise, often with such difficult and intimidating names that patients and doctors forgot to ask how and why. The name "became" the disease. The meaning of the word "diagnosis" changed. It did not mean understanding how and why anymore. It became the title of a list of symptoms and test results that matched most of the ones the patient presented with. It had become a code. A diagnosis could be entered into a computer and a list of medications that were covered by insurance companies for that specific code would appear on the screen. It also showed how many days of hospital stay were approved for that same code. What the doctor thought did not matter as much anymore.

The practice of medicine was looking a lot like the supermarkets that early on had impressed me so much. It was very evident that I wasn't the only one whose cells were forgetting their chemistry. The growth in the rates of depression was all around me. More and more patients were on antidepressants. Health news was full of reports on the rising epidemic of diseases connected to diet and lifestyle. And the financial news echoed with reports of the meteoric rise in the value of stock in pharmaceutical companies, especially the ones that had patented antidepressants. My specialty, heart disease, headed the list of problems, followed by cancer. The World Health Organization announced that these diseases occurred at higher rates in industrialized countries than in developing nations.

It didn't make sense. On one hand, science and technology were advancing in giant leaps. We had broken the genetic code, invented nanotechnology, and created robots that perform surgery. There was a false sense of security and hope that, sooner or later, medicine would discover the cure for everything. Yet, when I looked around, I saw that everybody was sick. Everyone was on medications. Judging by the results, our medical system was not working. The more technologically advanced we became, the sicker we got. We had not improved health on the planet or our planet's health. On the contrary, things were getting worse, sooner and faster.

Diseases seemed to affect younger and younger patients all the time. Obesity, type 2 diabetes, high blood pressure, and many other chronic diseases used to be seen primarily in the aging population. Now one in three American kids were overweight or obese, and the trend was growing. These statistics and trends were obtained by analyzing data from hospitals and doctors' offices, where patients are never asked about the bigger picture, and the small-picture inventory was lacking information as essential as diet. Apparently, there was no time for that.

At random times during my days of "factory line" medicine, my meditation teacher's words would ring in my ears, "Don't worry, don't hurry," interrupting the rush from patient to patient and bringing me into the present moment. I would suddenly remember to apply the same observation methodology in the clinic that I used in India. In this way, another picture started to emerge. I noticed a quieter, but even bigger problem, one that existed off the radar, that was not reported by the media, and had no clinical studies and research: a stream of people who did not have major health problems, yet were physically, mentally, and emotionally "off." Bloated, tired, itchy, moody, sneezy, constipated, foggy, swollen—it seemed as if most of my patients and friends had some type of disorder about to surface.

Curiously, the blood and other tests routinely ordered at a physical examination were absolutely normal. Without an explanation and reassured that nothing was really wrong by the normal test results, these people accepted their complaints as part of ordinary modern life, often justified as the wear and tear on our body parts, the expected result of aging. But left unattended, these conditions were the beginning of a more serious disorder. Looking at the patients' bigger picture, one would invariably find parallel social, financial, or emotional distress.

I kept searching for an answer, a diagnosis in the "old school" sense. What was making humanity so uncomfortable, unhappy, irritated, and sick? What was the bigger picture?

As above, so below. This universal rule guides the holistic thinking that is the backbone of most Eastern traditions of healing. To fully understand a cell, one has to understand the organism of which that cell is a part and how it relates to the other cells in it. In the school of meditation in India I learned to look at planet Earth as a living organism. According to this analogy, the rivers are its arteries, the forests its lungs, the mountain chains its ribs, and human beings, circulating by the billions, are one of the many types of cells that inhabit this organism. Humans were getting sick, but what about the planet, the organism they are a part of? That was also in the news, just not in the health section. In those days, it was starting to make headlines: global warming, "an inconvenient truth." The Earth had a fever.

A fever is a symptom that reveals there is something wrong somewhere. It is a nonspecific sign. Many different diseases can cause a fever as one of their symptoms. It is important to find out what exactly is causing it, so we can treat the real cause, not just bring the temperature down. In order to find the cause, doctors ask questions, observe, and order blood tests to see the circulating cells and also to study the chemicals that reveal the inner climate. With all the information gathered, a diagnosis can be made. In modern

Western cultures, because it's so common, cancer is on the "suspect" list when a fever persists. It is in everyone's mind even when getting a routine checkup. Very often, when I sit with patients to go over their tests results, before I get a chance to speak, they ask, "Doc, just tell me. Do I have cancer?" It is probably the most feared diagnosis.

Cancer cells are also cells that forgot how to do their chemistry. But cancer cells forgot how to do their math as well, and their geography, and their grammar, and even how to behave within a community. When you look at cancer cells under a microscope, you see cells that kill each other and every other cell in the neighborhood; they grow and reproduce unusually fast, disregarding the natural laws of space, population density, and food availability. They also have a tendency to travel to distant places and conquer new territories. When that happens, it's called *metastasis*, and it means the cancer has spread. Cancer cells eat different foods than healthy cells. The waste products they eliminate into the circulatory system are often toxic chemicals that affect the whole organism that hosts them. Cancer cells, like most cells, are microscopic, but size doesn't matter. Such a small organism can initiate an inner revolution that can kill the strongest of men and women.

These thoughts were on my mind as I searched for the answer to my question. Sometimes a diagnosis takes time. Many times, when someone is obsessed with a question, the answer comes at the least expected moment, when one is doing or seeing something seemingly unrelated. A sudden realization closes an inner loop, and an "Aha!" moment occurs, like an inner detonation that sends waves that can be felt all over the body.

This "Aha!" moment came for me soon after I started my detox program at We Care. The effects of eliminating toxins and the dulling mucus from my body lifted a cloud that had prevented me from seeing.

The planet has a fever. Random chemical analysis and laboratory tests of the planets' fluids and gases show something alarming. There are toxic chemicals everywhere. These chemicals are affecting everything and every other cell in this organism. The planet is in critical condition. If nothing changes, the prognosis is fatal in the short term.

One type of cell on the planet, the human cell, is behaving erratically, killing its own kind and every other type of cell. This cell has eating habits that are very different from those of all other cells. The human cell manufactures toxic chemicals that are mixed with food and used for many other functions as well as released into the circulation, through which they kill other cells even in distant places. The human cell reproduces fast and disregards the natural laws of population density, space, and food supply. Humans are cutting down all of Earth's trees and clogging up Earth's lungs. The balance has tipped: toxins, greenhouse gases among them, are accumulating faster than Earth's ability to neutralize and eliminate them. Toxicity is killing us and the planet. The planet has cancer, and we are it. This is what I call "another inconvenient truth."

My question was finally answered at the cellular level. My cells had never forgotten how to do their chemistry. They were actually desperately trying to do it. But the toxic chemicals I was consuming in my food and exposed to living in a large urban center such as New York had changed the inner climate. Many of these toxins were obstacles to normal cell functioning, causing irritation and inflammation. Toxins had damaged cells and tissues, and many systems had started to malfunction. My body's natural ability to heal itself was further weakened because the chemicals needed for cells to do their chemistry, the nutrients from foods, were no longer present in sufficient amounts.

Starting with my guts and going all the way to my brain, these changes presented as symptoms that matched two lists from the "diagnosis" menu, depression and irritable bowel syndrome. More chemicals were prescribed, which I refused to take. Instead, I had finally found a way to remove these obstacles and provide what was missing, so my cells could do their chemistry. That is what happened in my case, through detoxification and cleansing. I finally connected the dots.

From the way I was feeling and looking, I knew that my cells were getting straight A's in their chemistry reports. But I also knew that some of them had gone beyond and were not doing chemistry anymore—this was alchemy.

TOXICITY: THE MAKING OF A DIAGNOSIS

Doctors who are really good at finding the cause of symptoms are called "great diagnosticians." One such doctor once told me, "We usually end up finding what we are looking for, but we only look for what we already know."

The toxic attack we are under is so evident to me now. But during my training days in New York hospitals, despite suffering greatly and desperately looking for solutions, I never heard or read about global toxicity as a health hazard. I cannot understand how Western medicine continues to be blind to its existence and its contribution to disease. It was a revelation I stumbled upon outside of the hospital setting, and it allowed me to restore my own well-being beyond what I believed possible after all my study and years of training.

It's not surprising that I didn't know about this earlier. Toxicity continues to be a condition that modern medicine barely registers. When the word is used in hospital settings, it describes cases of acute poisoning (such as when a child accidentally ingests hazardous chemicals or someone takes too much of a certain prescription drug) or getting off alcohol or drugs. And when asked about detox from the Clean perspective, many physicians discard it as quackery. Doctors who are skeptical about the value of detox programs such as Clean will argue that there is nothing in "the literature" to support it. What they mean is that when you search the medical database, you find no scientific studies or published research on such detox programs.

Databases only contain what the editors decide to include, making them biased toward Western medical studies with Western protocols. This perpetuates and strengthens the status quo, which too often discards valuable approaches like chelation as anecdotal or quackery. Furthermore, the research game is biased before it begins. The cost of large-scale double-controlled placebo studies makes pharmaceutical companies the only ones that can afford to fund them. If there is no wonder drug with revenue potential in question, there are usually no funds for research. It is not good for business to prove that vegetables and fruits can be the most powerful medicine. But the new field of Functional Medicine is rapidly filling this void by validating a new database of its own design, taking into consideration the multidimensional matrix of influences that play a role in health. Functional Medicine is the perfect blend of Eastern thinking and Western technology, and the results are great.

Toxicity is not a disease or one specific symptom. It is a condition that exists right now, one we are responsible for and one that is threatening the planet and all life. I use the word *toxicity* to describe the wider, low-grade state that, to one degree or another, everyone who breathes today's air, eats today's food, and lives in today's cities, suburbs, or rural areas is experiencing inside.

Toxicity can manifest as many different symptoms. It can also show no symptoms at all. Regardless of whether you notice it or not, there is no escaping its reach. And to different degrees, everyone is paying the price.

Toxicity, as I present it to you in Clean, is a problem that reveals an evolutionary glitch. Evolution is what happens as organisms adapt and overcome obstacles and threats. Driven by the instinct for survival, organisms grow wings, develop ridiculously long necks, or learn how to transform certain chemicals into others. The human body has developed a very effective and incredibly sophisticated system of organs and functions that complement each other in the effort to achieve one sole purpose—to detoxify. Somehow our physical body has evolved just right. But that evolutionary state must be helped by our thinking and behavior.

The evolutionary glitch I am referring to stems from the fact that, despite an exponential increase in the exposure to and damage by toxins in modern life, our modern "lifestyle" has slowed down the single most important evolutionary tool that was so intelligently designed for our bodies. Our thinking and habits need to evolve or our bodies will die of dust while we hold a state-of-the-art vacuum cleaner in our hands. To help you understand how to plug in and use that vacuum cleaner effectively is the purpose of Clean.

Toxins that cannot be eliminated in a timely manner remain in circulation, causing irritation and damage. Cells and tissues trap these toxins and coat them with mucus in an attempt to buffer the irritation. This survival mechanism, like inflammation, is life-saving for a while, but can turn fatal when turned on continuously for a prolonged time.

In Eastern traditions, one of the first things practitioners check is the ability of the body to eliminate toxins. Indian Ayurvedic doctors or Chinese medicine practitioners immediately hunt for clues to toxic-waste retention or accumulation. They look for signs like dullness in the skin, white coating on the tongue, or gray, yellow, or pink tones in the whites of the eyes. They want to know if you have regular bowel movements, urinate a lot or a little, and when and how much you sweat. Their traditions, thousands of years old, consider the ability to detoxify—to eliminate toxic waste and toxic thought and emotion—as the "root" source of your physical and mental health. The loss of this ability helps explain why you might have allergies, headaches, constipation, nightmares, fertility problems, and unidentifiable pain among a host of other ailments.

Toxicity is not a new problem. Long before we added the burden of human-made chemicals to our bodies, toxic buildup could occur from eating too much, especially too many heavy or hard to digest foods, and eating under stress. In Europe and America, there were early proponents of cleansing who taught that damage to the intestinal tract from overeating and ingesting refined foods was the main cause of disease affecting civilized, affluent society. They called the condition that resulted "autointoxication." Some of them, like the famous turn-of-the-century naturopath Arnold Ehret, put his patients on a "mucus-less" diet to promote health and longevity, which was his form of the Elimination Diet, which you will experience as part of Clean. These pioneers and all those after them who taught natural healing methods understood that the digestive and detoxification systems are well engineered to keep us healthy, but they must be kept in balance. As you will discover, even basic foods, when not well digested and eliminated, can create a polluted inner state. This can then harm the whole balance of health—even before human-made chemicals enter the picture.

Western medicine had this understanding in the past. Many older people will tell you how their family doctor would dose them with castor oil when they were sick in bed, because a big expulsion of toxins could be enough to alleviate the sickness and start recovery. Colonic rooms used to be standard in hospitals at the turn of the century. In the rush to make medical care more "advanced" and more profitable, basic wisdom—and low-cost, drug-free protocols—got dropped. But they're needed now more than ever. If you live in today's environment but never pay attention to good detoxification, you end up like a tree that has been growing by a busy highway for years, absorbing smog, dirty water, and the stress of loud cars going by. You end up polluted and wilted, with dull, spindly leaves.

No matter how you look at it, understanding what toxins are, where they are, how they affect your health, and what to do about them in a safe way may save your life, and if things don't change dramatically soon, this understanding may be needed to save life on Earth, and ultimately Earth's life.

WHAT IS A TOXIN?

A toxin is something that interferes with normal physiology and negatively impacts bodily function. Toxins are of many different kinds, with totally different qualities, from an infinite number of different sources; just as varied are the complex mechanisms by which they cause irritation and damage.

Some toxins, known as endotoxins, are waste products from the normal activity of cells. Uric acid, ammonia, lactic acid, and homocysteine fall in this category. When these toxins build up, they cause diseases. Some are very specific; for example, when uric acid lingers, it causes gout.

Exotoxins, or xenobiotics, are human-made toxins that we are exposed to intentionally or inadvertently. Thousands of chemicals are being invented every year.

These chemicals, alone or in combination, may cause disruption of the normal cell function. Throughout the following chapters, Clean will continually point out the toxins you need to be aware of (including specific names), where they are, and how to measure them. It will also describe how these toxins affect your health and what you can do to prevent disease or repair the damage that has been already done

WHERE ARE TOXINS LOCATED?

The Four Skins

Studies now show that every person living today carries measurable levels of several hundred synthetic chemicals in his or her body. These contaminants did not exist prior to the twentieth century and have no role in our body chemistry. It is safe to assume that all of us are burdened with a toxic load from exposure to synthetic substances: pesticides, phthalates, mercury, trans-fatty acids, benzene, trihalomethanes. Exotoxins have names scary enough to make any smart person want to avoid them. The evidence is now undeniable that what we don't know *can* hurt us. It's estimated that the average American comes into contact with thousands of potentially harmful chemicals every day.

To understand the way we are exposed to toxins, it is useful to imagine four layers separating our inner chemistry from the rest of the universe, as if we had four skins.

THE FIRST SKIN

The first skin is what separates our blood, tissues, and organs from the outside world; it is the outermost edge of our physical bodies, just one layer of cells thick. To the naked eye, it may seem like a barrier, deceptively leading to a sense of separation, even protection. But under the microscope, things become less clear, since the first skin is in constant motion, selecting from the environment what to reject and what to actively capture and absorb. It also discards to the outside what we don't want or need inside anymore. The first skin uses two types of cells to form our body surfaces, depending on the location.

Epithelial cells. We see epithelial cells (dry, tough) at a simple glance. They form what we commonly call skin. When this part of our first skin gets sick, we visit a dermatologist. The major source of toxins entering through this skin are the cosmetics and toiletries we use. Think of everything you rub or spray onto your skin on purpose. Do you read the labels? You should think of cosmetics as food. Ideally, you should only use cosmetics that you feel safe eating, because, just like food, they will end up circulating in your blood. Your choice of products should be guided more by the ingredients list than the promised effect. This information is no secret. Doctors use creams, gels, and ointments to deliver many prescription drugs into the blood through the skin.

Dyes, fragrances, foaming agents, heavy metals as stabilizers and texturizers, tanners, inks, alcohols, and hundreds of other potential poisons are frequently included in cosmetic formulas. Nail products, hair products, deodorants—all the ordinary products in your bathroom cabinet and makeup kit as well as the ones in your neighborhood beauty salon and nail spa have chemical compounds that don't exist in nature. They can cause irritation, allergies, and sensitivities, just like food. Endocrine-system disruptions are problems linked to a group of chemicals found in skin and hair products called parabens. Many deodorants contain aluminum to stop you from sweating. They give you a double whammy, introducing one more chemical into the circulation while shutting down your pores, which were originally designed to eliminate toxins.

The water we shower with is absorbed through the skin and ends up in our circulatory systems, just like the water we drink. Most city-supplied water has some amount of chlorine, which was used upstream to prevent bacteria from growing. It makes for a bacteria-free shower, but contributes to bacterial genocide in the intestines. Recent reports reveal that your shower and tap water may contain increasingly detectable levels of most of the popular prescription medications such as antidepressants, antibiotics, hormones, and immunosuppressants.

This skin is also in contact with the air around us. And many toxins carried in the air affect the other type of cell used for the first skin.

Mucosal cells. Mucosal cells (wet, soft) form the walls of the first skin in areas that are hidden from sight without using instruments. Many of my patients think of these areas as inside their bodies, but technically this type of first skin separates in and out as much as the epidermis. When we breathe in, air gushes down the trachea and bronchi, finally hitting the wall of alveoli, where mucosal cells are quick to absorb oxygen, since it is such a precious commodity. You are probably aware of airborne toxins like car, factory, and cigarette smoke, but has it ever occurred to you that breathing your hair spray could be worse than second-hand smoke?

The urethra, vagina, and uterus are also lined with mucosa. There are toxins in products used on these areas.

Of all the "first skins," the one coating the inside of the digestive tract is the largest and busiest; it is the most important site of exposure to the toxins of modern life. The chemicals of modern life enter our circulatory system starting with our mouths. In the past, silver amalgam fillings were frequently prepared with mercury. It takes many years for them to leak into your blood. Toothpaste, mouth rinses, breath sprays, and other dental products introduce toxic chemicals as well.

The intestines, a twenty-five-foot-long tube that connects the stomach to the anus, has two distinct sections. The small intestine is about twenty feet long and an inch and a half in diameter. The large intestine is wider, but shorter (about five feet). When food enters the digestive tube, it is broken down in small pieces and absorbed into our circulatory system by the cells that form the intestinal wall. The wall of this tube is not smooth like the surface of the pages of this book. In order to increase the surface area for the purpose of maximizing absorption of nutrients, the walls have folds (villi), which in turn, have folds of their own (microvilli). If we opened and completely stretched out an average intestinal tube, its surface area would cover a tennis court.

It is said that a person who lives eighty years digests twenty-five tons of food in his or her lifetime.

Understanding food as a source of toxicity through our first skin is vital, and we will cover it in detail in the coming pages. Besides food, everything else that enters the tube is absorbed, such as prescription and over-the-counter medications. Drugs in America today may be causing more damage than the problems they are supposed to solve. Not only are many toxic chemicals themselves, but they also contribute to nutrient depletion as a side effect.

I see common drugs affecting patients every day. Beta blockers, used to manage cardiac arrhythmia and high blood pressure, deplete the body of coenzyme Q10 (needed to maintain heart functioning, normal blood pressure, and energy levels). Statin drugs, used to lower cholesterol, deplete coenzyme Q10, calcium (needed to regulate bone strength, blood clotting, and cell rigidity), and beta-carotene (a vision and immunity booster). Oral contraceptives, used to prevent pregnancy, deplete vitamin B2 (needed for eye, nerve, skin health), vitamin B6 (helps avoid depression, cardiovascular disease, sleep disorders), vitamin B12 (needed to prevent anemia, weakness), and zinc (immune system booster, sense of taste and smell).

Imagine what happens to your nutritional status when, like the average senior citizen today, you're taking up to ten prescription drugs daily. Even if, to manage an ongoing condition, you are simply taking two or three, they all get in line to be processed out by the liver, while they continue to prevent absorption of essential nutrients. (For a full list of prescription drugs and the depletions they cause, please see appendix "Prescription Drugs and Nutritional Depletion.")

Prescription drugs have important uses, and there is a time and a place for them. I prefer to prescribe them as a "bridge"—something to help the patient transition while we work together on boosting the body's own ability to heal.

THE SECOND SKIN

What I call the "second skin" is the layer that we put right on top of our epidermis. It includes clothing and everything used to clean, process, color, and perfume it. Today most of the material we press against our bodies is more heavily sprayed with pesticide than our foods. Growing cotton uses 25 percent of the world's pesticides and 10 percent of its insecticides, which get into the ground, water, and air, not to mention vast amounts of chemical fertilizers. (The bulk of chemicals from cotton get into us through food, via the cottonseed fed to dairy cows and used in junk food.) Add to that the petroleum-based synthetic clothes we have become accustomed to wearing—acrylic, nylon, polyester, and so forth—which harm the environment and can leach toxins into us too.

Wearing synthetic clothes typically also inhibits the evaporation of fluids that your skin releases, and they get reabsorbed. (In addition, habits that kept humans healthy in the past—like sweat rooms and saunas—are missing from modern life. You will be encouraged to include these as part of the Clean program.) Many textiles are finished with a formaldehyde resin to make them crease-resistant, waterproof, and shrink-proof—especially sheets and bedding made of a polyester-cotton mix. Sleep in a cloud of formaldehyde, and insomnia, not to mention headaches, asthma, and skin rashes, can likely result. Children's sleepwear, meanwhile, is legally required to contain toxic fire retardants.

Now consider the new trend of wearing plastic clogs constantly, not to mention spending all summer in flip-flops. (If plastics leach out of sun-warmed bottles into water, what are plastic shoes doing to your sweaty feet?) Then there are the detergents, highly toxic dryer sheets, and, worse, dry-cleaning fluids used to care for all these second-skin products. You only have to look at a bottle of supersized, bleach-enhanced detergent or take a whiff of the suit inside your cleaner's plastic wrapping to get a sense of this invisible source of exposure. The dry-cleaning chemical perchloroethylene is known to cause liver, kidney, and neurological damage as a result of both short- and long-term exposure.

THE THIRD SKIN

The next skin, slightly farther out, is our living-space environment—our homes and workplaces. It is calculated that one-third of the planet's pollution comes from the chemicals we use to manufacture the materials for building and the carbon gases generated in doing so. Included in that is everything we use for furnishing, decorating, cleaning, and maintaining our homes. According to the Environmental Protection Agency, indoor air is more polluted than outdoor air, due largely to all the emissions from furnishings, paints, foam, insulators, fire retardants, veneers, and flooring as well as dust, dander, and sometimes cigarette smoke. Synthetic wall-to-wall carpeting is loaded with chemicals.

Asbestos and lead may make the headlines as household toxins that must be identified and removed, but seemingly less dangerous things like shower curtains emit their own poisonous compounds. That new-shower-curtain smell, just like the "new car smell" that many people love, is a chemical off-gassing from the PVC (polyvinyl chloride) plastic, commonly referred to as vinyl. It is one of the most hazardous consumer products ever created. One recent study showed that elevated levels of dangerous airborne toxins from shower curtains can persist for more than a month—a good reason to buy some organic cotton ones.

Think of everything we use to clean our living, working, and even driving environments. Plenty has been written about the downside of chemical-filled household cleaning products and how the toxins in them are linked to cancer, immune system disorders, liver damage, and many other very common health issues. But you don't even need to study the scientific findings telling you that bleach has been linked to reproductive problems in men and learning and behavioral problems in children, that the fumes given off by carpet cleaners can cause cancer and liver damage, or that air "fresheners" spew poisons into the living room. Just use your common sense. Anything with a smell that can trigger a headache is causing a disturbance in the cells and should be avoided. And a combination of these products used at the same time? They're going to react together as you inhale them and cause even greater damage. (Just because something is inhaled instead of eaten doesn't make it harmless. Molecules breathed into the lungs enter the bloodstream and circulate around the body too. That's why spending hours in a recently painted room or a photo lab or working with glues and dyes all add to the toxic load your body must process and dispose of.)

It's easy to get started replacing toxic cleaning products, because trendy new eco-companies provide green cleaning products at a friendly price. But one thing we don't often consider: the traditional cleaning products that boast of their power to kill "99.9 percent of germs" or that advertise themselves as "antibacterial" are slaughtering the good bacteria your intestines are working hard to nurture in order to protect you—which you will read about later. Meanwhile you lose your resistance to the bad bacteria from lack of contact. More than anything, reducing exposure to toxins in the third skin is what green architecture is all about. Make informed consumer choices.

THE FOURTH SKIN

The fourth skin is a gigantic layer that ends at the edges of our planetary atmosphere. It contains an innumerable number of different toxins, many of them by-products of agriculture, industry, and transportation. Emissions from cars, trucks, and planes pour out into the air. Where you live can make it worse, of course. Those who live by highways or near factories are subject to more intense exposure. Recent research indicates that a few hours of exposure to heavy air pollution increases the rate of heart attacks.

Heavy metals such as cadmium, mercury, arsenic, chromium, and lead compounds, which are emitted into our environment and consumer products, can accumulate in fatty tissues when they exist in high enough concentrations and over prolonged periods of time. They affect and disrupt many brain functions, since they have a high affinity for fat, which makes up 90 percent of our brain. Some, like mercury, can be deposited in soils or surface waters, where they are taken up by plants, which are then ingested by animals. Mercury accumulates in greater concentrations as you go up the food chain. When people and animals at the top of the food chain eat fish or meat contaminated with mercury, they get exposed to concentrations that are much higher than those in the water, air, or soil.

Here in the fourth skin we find toxins in the form of electromagnetic frequencies (EMFs). The radiation from power lines, cell phones and headsets, computers, and all the electrical objects that surround us daily is considered by some in the scientific and healing worlds to cause the same sensitivity and symptoms that chemical toxins do. Research links the modern bombardment with even low-level frequencies to brain cancer and miscarriages. Today there is a lot of discussion of the dangers of cell phones. Since there is as yet no consensus regarding the dangers, it makes sense to be cautious and limit their use to situations in which a land line is not available.

CHAPTER FOUR

Modern Food Exposed: We Are What We Eat

The source of chemical exposure that we have the most intimate contact with is our food. Food is one of the most important commodities to any living organism, but humans take it to a whole different level than any other organism. Our lives revolve around food. We celebrate with food, we mourn with food. Many people spend the most significant moments with family and friends sitting at a table, eating and drinking. At the most basic, obvious, and literal level, we are what we eat. Food provides the materials for the construction of our body's architecture. Food becomes us.

Food determines many other aspects of our lives, and these change with time. Early on, humans would gather around abundant sources of food and water. These locations turned into villages, towns, and cities. The maps of early civilizations were drawn with a fork.

We used to pick our food from trees, the soil, and the shorelines and hunt or fish for the rest. We used to eat whenever we could. Food would go bad without refrigerators. The modern food system has, in only a few decades, profoundly changed the way we get, or don't get, our nutrients.

Now we buy food in modern supermarkets. It is loaded with chemicals that alone or in combination can cause disease. Ninety percent of the products in the supermarkets come in some kind of container. In order to extend shelf life outside a fridge, these food-like products are loaded with preservatives—chemicals that kill bacteria. Most products also contain additives to give them the most attractive color, smell, taste, and texture possible, so we will be tempted to buy and eat them. The remaining 10 percent of edible items in supermarkets—produce, fish, meat, and dairy products—are put through plenty of unnatural steps as well. The dietary expression of global toxicity has an even darker side. Stories come out every day about contaminated food sources in our supermarkets and fast-food chains. We hear about potentially lethal bacteria scares and nationwide meat and vegetable recalls, directly caused by the intensive way we mass-produce foods. (This has led to the practice of irradiating more foods—which zaps nutritional value out of your bagged spinach and leaves you with little more than a bunch of limp leaves.)

Recently, a fish farm was fined and a fish recall ordered when it was discovered that the fish were being fed recalled dog food. Think of that: what is not good enough for your dog to eat ends up becoming the building blocks that create *you*—and at a much higher price than dog food. When it's safer to share your pet's meals than to buy the fish that the health experts all tell you to consume, you have to conclude there's a madness behind the quest for cheapness and convenience, one that, if we don't stop it, may end up sending us to the hospital (and have you ever seen the food there?).

For this reason, one of the most powerful ways you can reduce your exposure to toxins and increase the nutrient content of your food is to spend more on foods with safer pedigrees—when possible, buy fresh foods from local sources. Imported foods have to be transported, and in the process of getting from field, farm, or body of water to your plate, your food is exposed to a chemical mix that includes fertilizers, pesticides, and insecticides (to kill the bugs that might compete for the food), hormones (to fatten animals faster or make them produce more milk), and antibiotics (to prevent animals with weak immune systems from getting infected). It goes through invisible processes like radiation

Overexposure: Diet and Kids

Sometimes the impact of the modern diet makes itself known in alarming ways. Unfortunately, toxins take the biggest toll on children, whose small body size means they're more affected by everyday amounts. When patients are resistant to the idea of using organic foods, I tell them about my friend and colleague Tina, with whom I worked in Palm Springs. A dynamo of a mom who has won national bodybuilding championships and competed in Eco-Challenges, she has two beautiful daughters. She presented me with one of my earliest toxicity cases.

Several years ago, she called me extremely worried because her daughter, Annie, age seven at the time, had gotten her period and was developing breasts and pubic hair. I immediately sent her to the best pediatric endocrinologist I could find to rule out the possibility of a brain tumor in her daughter's hypophysis, the gland that regulates the sex hormones. After no tumor was found, the specialist, still confounded by this alarmingly early development, wanted to start her on a chemotherapy drug to stop her sex-hormone production.

We decided to look for an alternative and quickly realized Annie wasn't alone. Her problem was another silent crisis in American health. The chemicals in everyday food, especially the hormones in our animal products, were mimicking sex hormones that her body shouldn't have had until years later. She was experiencing artificially induced development—a sign of inner chaos that was not only psychologically harmful, but would throw the whole balance of her health into disarray. Immediately Tina stopped buying anything that was not 100 percent USDA-approved organic. Her grocery bill tripled, but it was worth it. Annie's condition reversed: her periods stopped, and her breasts and pubic hair did not develop further until she hit her teens.

This story is an extreme case because it affected such a young person, but it shows how the exposure to toxins from food is changing our bodies at every level and how the body can self-correct after a total dietary change. It also shows how the invasive medical treatment prescribed would have exposed Annie to potentially lethal toxicity from chemotherapy drugs—without correcting the root problem.

(X-raying to eliminate bacteria, which also kills nutrients), pasteurization (extreme heat to kill pathogens—along with helpful enzymes), hydrogenation (altering fats and oils to make them shelf stable, a condition that harms your own cells when you eat them), and even cosmetic procedures like waxing (to make the fruits look nicer in the market).

The technological processes used today for "safety," cosmetic, productivity, and convenience purposes turn much of what we eat into poison. With the thought, "If it's good for the baby, it must be good for us," we started drinking milk and using it to make a hundred other foods. We became the only mammals that drink milk after we stop nursing from our mother's breast. And we go even farther—we steal the milk from different species. It's like putting jet fuel in a motorcycle; it damages the engine. Worse, now that milk is full of hormones and antibiotics, a questionable argument becomes undeniable. Milk is poisoning us.

My own story, of arriving in North American supermarket culture and getting sick, is far from unusual. In fact, anthropologists show how it has happened around the globe, many times over. Scientific studies show that when immigrants exchange traditional, local diets, full of vegetables picked from the field (with nutrient-filled soil still on them) and home-raised animal protein, for the American diet, full of sugar, processed foods, and chemical drinks, their obesity, diabetes, and heart-disease rates increase unusually fast—in a single generation.

Patients are often surprised when I tell them that some of the most common toxins are the foods on their daily plate. Wheat, dairy products, and eggs as well as corn and soy are allergic triggers in a large number of people. This is partly because of the way these foods are produced today, with chemicals, antibiotics, and lots of pesticides, but also partly because the human intestinal tract didn't evolve to process them in mass quantity. Dealing with large quantities of them was not part of our original design.

Water is another source of toxicity today. Our tap water is treated with chlorine to kill microscopic organisms instantly—which means in the case of large-sized organisms like humans the damage just takes a little longer. Fluoride is added to many public water systems ostensibly to strengthen teeth—but it's a known toxin now linked to problems with the thyroid, kidneys, central nervous system, and skeletal system, including cancers (not to mention lower IQs).

But there's much more in our ordinary H_2O than that. Carcinogens (cancer-causing compounds) from industrial toxins in the air and runoff from other wastes in

Toxic Symphony

It's important to know that: (1) toxins tend to bio-accumulate, meaning that they build up in our tissues and cells more quickly than they are eliminated, and (2) toxins work alone and in synergy with each other. Scientists admit we are fundamentally ignorant of the way the thousands of chemicals we're exposed to interact once inside our tissues or cells. But we know that synergy—two or more things coming together and creating an effect that is bigger than the sum of their parts—is happening. This means that in this new world in which chemicals pervade our food, air, and water supplies, assurances of safety from official sources about one ingredient or another are almost useless. There is never a moment when we're exposed to a single chemical in isolation. It is an orchestra, not a single instrument.

Multiple toxins are already combining in our bodies, altering and shifting our inner environments in ways that we're only just starting to figure out. One basic reaction should be a red flag alerting us to how much disturbance must be going on daily: we know that fluoride, the chemical in toothpaste and many water supplies, actually depletes stores of the essential nutrient iodine from the body. Researchers, meanwhile, present new evidence of how cocktails of pesticides mixed together in rivers and lakes are infinitely more lethal to frogs and fish than a single dose of one pesticide alone could ever be. More evidence is coming out every day about the ways that harmful chemical reactions are happening throughout the body in thousands of small ways at the same time.

the modern world make it through water-treatment facilities in trace amounts and into our tap water. Drinking water disinfection by-product (DBP) is a newly identified danger, formed when the chemicals used for disinfecting drinking water react with natural organic matter in the source water. And our water is even medicating us more. A recent study showed that 41 million Americans drink water contaminated with antidepressants, hormones, heart medications, and other prescription and over-the-counter medications that have made it through the water-treatment system. It's not just in the kitchen. The city-supplied water in our showers and bathtubs has equal potential to add to the toxic load, because we absorb more water through our skin via bathing and showering than through drinking.

We've also strayed from natural, simpler ways of packaging food. Instead of buying raw materials from a greengrocer or butcher that are then wrapped in paper or carried in our baskets, we buy food that comes in plastic packaging. This can leach chemicals into our food, which we then consume. This human-made mix includes chemical compounds known as phthalates, one of the most abundant modern chemicals produced today, designed to give certain plastics their rigidity. Though we come across phthalates in multiple ways all day long, they're especially prevalent in water and beverage bottles. And though they cross over into our foods and drinks in micro amounts, their effects can build up. The chemistry of phthalates mimics the chemistry of hormones, which are the message-carrying agents of the body. When levels of it build up in us over time, one result is that hormone function may be disturbed. This can be like air-traffic control suddenly going down at the airport. Signals get scrambled, and our normal functioning starts to crash—without any obvious cause. Now that two hormonally linked cancers, breast and prostate cancer, are on a rapid rise and the number of thyroid disorders is going through the roof, toxic specialists are pointing the finger at phthalates among other toxic causes.

Another chemical, styrene, seeps into foods when it out-gases from food containers. Studies showed 100 percent of a group of people tested had it in their fat. Imagine how this load accumulates: a steak at the supermarket is packed on a polystyrene tray and wrapped in plastic wrap; then you grill it, which blackens it (blackening food has cancer-causing potential) and put some additive-filled sauce on it. Delicious.

Bisphenol-A (BPA) is another chemical used to make hard plastic containers like drinking bottles and to line cans of foods. When enough of it builds up in the body, it is thought to promote cancer.

Toxic chemicals are only one of the reasons why eating food, such a life-giving practice for the rest of nature, has turned deadly for us.

YOU EAT WHAT YOU ARE

There's another side of food-based toxicity that keeps you stuck and sick. The standard American diet, with its quantities of refined grains and sugars and engineered, processed foods, has also created a roller-coaster ride of cravings and energy swings—a key factor in both contributing to and maintaining our modern toxic states. I frequently ask my patients if they know what the phrase "You are what you eat" means. Most say yes—the quality of the food you eat directly translates into the quality of your body. To put it more specifically, it means that the food you choose to eat becomes the building blocks of your architecture; the compounds that the body makes from food are what it uses to build your bones, muscles, tissues, and even the molecules and enzymes that fund your chemistry. You literally are what you eat.

Andres, a dear friend and patient once surprised me. He said, "Doc, the opposite is also true. You eat what you are. When I was puffed up, sluggish, and emotionally dulled from toxicity, I craved the foods that gave me an initial jolt of energy, a boost. But after the rush came the crash, and the cycle started all over again. After the Clean program I am craving really healthy foods."

I told Andres that craving toxic food is a classic sign of a toxic state. Toxins that cannot be dealt with immediately and continue in the circulatory system are soon trapped in the tissues and covered with mucus. This is the way cells defend themselves. Mucus has a dense and sticky quality; it resonates with and attracts dense, toxic thoughts and emotions. The reverse is also true, that dense thoughts and emotions promote mucus production in the tissues.

Instead, by enhancing the elimination of mucus during Clean, you will stop craving the foods that perpetuate it. As you provide the nutrients that your cells are desperately waiting for, your natural ability to regenerate and heal is reactivated and your adrenal strength is restored. Instead of dense, "dead," processed foods you will acquire a taste for live foods, which still carry the energy of life. These were exactly what Andres was craving by the end of his third week on Clean.

DIET IN AMERICA: FROM FAD TO SAD

Anywhere I go, as soon as people find out what I do, they always ask, "Doctor, what should I eat?" Americans are obsessed with finding the right diet formula. Since 1990, the year I moved to New York, I have witnessed many theories and fads that swept the country, reshaped the industry, and left more casualties than all of the wars ever fought by the United States added together!

First was the war on fat. America's full frontal attack on fat redefined life in America. With doctors and the media in agreement, the population was convinced that fat was a hidden weapon of mass destruction, so it was eliminated from every single product in the supermarket. The food industry was having a party. The supermarkets were inundated with everything fat-free, you name it. Even the impossible, fat-free butter, endorsed by cardiologists! The caloric void that fats left was filled with carbs. "Lean" was the buzzword, but not the result. Instead, Americans became the fattest people in the world.

At Lenox Hill Hospital, during my fellowship, the casualties of this war kept our cardiac catheterization lab open 24/7 reopening coronary arteries with balloons and stents to abort or avoid a heart attack. During one of those long nights, walking alongside a gurney on the way from the emergency room to the angioplasty room, I heard my patient laughing so hard, his oxygen mask flew off his face. Before putting his mask back on, I asked him what was so funny. He said, "I just changed my favorite phrase from 'I can't believe it's not butter' to 'I wish it had been butter'!" Finding humor in tragedy sometimes carried me through those long nights on call. It also reminded me how believing in the latest product invented can be dangerous, even if it's approved by the FDA and endorsed by cardiologists.

Before the wave of heart attacks slowed down, America found a new enemy, carbohydrates. It was war all over again, just as vicious and supported by most authorities. Getting leaner was not about eating lean foods, as we once thought; it was about eating "sugar-free." The calories missing after eliminating carbs were replaced with extra protein, not exactly by accident. High-protein, low-carbohydrate diets had been in use in America for a long time. Bodybuilders figured out early on that if you eat mostly protein, your muscles will grow faster and bigger. Bodybuilders are the leanest people not by birth, but by choice, great effort, and tons of protein. So to imitate them off went America on a rampage of consuming fish, chicken, steak, eggs, and cottage cheese (low-fat).

Years back, when I started my search to overcome depression, I knew only one thing for sure: being in shape helps. Before moving to New York, as a tae kwon do competitor I was in tiptop shape. I remembered clearly that everything was better in that state. I decided to force myself to run, and after a month I was running one hour every day. I avoided desserts and candy and drank more water than ever in my life. I got skinny fast, but except in my legs, my muscles were gone and my skin was saggy. I wanted to get toned and ripped. I wanted a six-pack, so I hired a personal trainer who had one. He had the knowledge of the bodybuilders. He turned me on to many books, magazines, and products all created to assist the body in building muscle and burning fat. We lifted weights four days a week, did cardio two days a week, and rested one. One day every two weeks, I was allowed to splurge on pizza and ice cream. I was such a dedicated student that I beat his prediction about the time it would take me to look like him by a month. And in a graduation ceremony of sorts, he passed on to me the secret weapon, *The Opus Diet.*

The book was written by Dan Duchaine, himself a bodybuilder, who noticed that a high-protein, low-carb diet would only take him so far. There was that last fat reserve that seemed impossible to burn. In competition, the bodybuilder with the least fat wins. Duchaine, determined to understand how to do it, studied physiology, endocrinology, and metabolism with such passion that he became an authority on those subjects.

His greatest discovery came from observing sick people. Poorly controlled diabetics develop a condition known in medicine as *ketoacidosis.* The lack of insulin prevents the glucose in the blood from entering the cells to be used as fuel for energy. The body has a temporary survival trick to buy time. It converts fat into ketone bodies, which are similar to glucose in that they can be used as fuel in cells, but their molecular composition resembles alcohol. The reason they are only a temporary solution is that they eventually make the blood so acid it is deadly. Ketoacidosis is a life-threatening medical emergency.

But patients who had repeated episodes of ketoacidosis were some of the leanest people Duchaine had ever seen, and he wanted to recreate this condition. Eating only protein and fat, no carbs, was his magic formula. He would go for as long as he could without carbs, allowing his body to turn fat into ketone bodies. Then, to keep from entering a critical state, he would eat some carbs to stabilize his blood acidity. Once it was stabilized, he would repeat the process. And it worked.

Duchaine knew the risk of death when eating this way. He knew well what he was dealing with, and he was willing to accept the consequences. But when the Atkins diet exploded all over the world, I don't think the majority of its followers knew what they were getting into. They still don't. The Atkins diet works; it is guaranteed to make you fit in your bathing suit by beach time. What it doesn't guarantee is that you will be alive to enjoy it. Ketoacidosis or not, high animal-protein content in our diet is acidifying, contributing to inflammation in general and to cardiovascular disease, cancer, renal insufficiency, gout, and osteoporosis in particular.

After this whole experience, whenever people ask me what they should eat, I first ask them, "What are you eating for?" If you are eating to get lean, fast, Atkins is your best choice, but your worst choice if what you want is radiant health and longevity.

When we finally realized that eliminating one of the three basic food categories (carbs, proteins, fats) was not going to work, more reasonable and safer fads, such as the Zone, South Beach, and Body for Life, came and went without as much press as their predecessors. Throughout the rise and fall of the fads, always in the background, as if pretending not to be there, was the U.S. government's food pyramid. It shows the different groups of foods and the number of servings per day that are considered healthy. The only thing I have to say about it is that it all starts with a lie; it turns out the pyramid is really a triangle.

Fads come and go; they often don't survive because they have no lasting value to impart to followers. Some dietary trends, however—those based on sound information and with lasting value—turn into movements. They are often born from the experience of someone who shares and inspires others to benefit from the discoveries made. Bonds are generated and communities are born. There are many Web communities that support these movements; they organize gatherings, lectures, and conventions as well as sell products and services. Movements can affect the country's economy as much as fads. Some of these movements are worth learning about.

The raw-food movement explains that it is not healthy to cook your food. Cooking destroys the enzymes in raw foods that are necessary for their digestion. A famous experiment I heard about made me fully respect the theories behind it. In the early 1900s, Dr. Francis Pottage conducted an experiment in California. He kept two groups of cats separated, living in identical environmental conditions, except for one difference. One group was fed raw meat and milk. The second group was fed the same amount of the same quality meat and milk, only cooked. After some time, the cats on raw food were healthy and thriving. The cats on cooked foods developed various diseases, such as cancer, arthritis, diabetes, and others—all diseases we see often in humans.

In my personal experience, eating only raw foods for a period of time is a great way to detox less intensely than juicing or water fasting. But after some time I myself could not sustain it. I was strongly drawn to eat cooked foods again, which invariably made me feel better. I do recommend that all my patients increase the percentage of raw foods in their daily diet. Small increases in percentage of foods eaten raw have proven to have significant benefits in lowering blood pressure and cholesterol naturally. The tenets of the raw-food movement are presented as the solution for a healthy body as well as a healthy planet. Shifting our habits to eating only raw foods would imply a total redesign of life as we know it, adherents explain, and will solve global warming, global toxicity, global hunger, and many other problems of modern life.

The live-food movement takes the ideas of the raw-food movement to another level. Simply being raw is not enough—food has to carry the energy of life. It cannot be eaten too long after picking or the energy of life will no longer be present. Seeds and nuts must be soaked to initiate the process of germination, before which the seed is inert, without any life energy.

Vegetarianism is the rare case of a dietary movement that people join for a whole host of reasons that have little to do with food, including religious and political ones. Still, whatever their motivation, they all reinforce each other, and the number of vegetarians is growing. Vegetarians eat both raw and cooked plants. Many vegetarians have to quit after some time, or they begin to look really unhealthy. Dr. Gabriel Cousens explains in his book *Conscious Eating* that becoming a healthy vegetarian is not as simple as having a salad for lunch and one for dinner. Certain nutrients are harder to get from plants, such as the B vitamins. There are ways around it, such as including fermented foods, so that all the needed nutrients can be obtained from a vegetarian diet. He explains that many people making the change to vegetarianism need to do so gradually. Dr. Dean Ornish was the first cardiologist to prove that blockages in the coronary arteries disappeared after switching to a vegetarian diet and meditating. He opened the door for modern medicine to begin to give food choices the importance they really deserve.

When it comes to diet, America is stuck in the wild, wild West. There are a thousand other theories that don't qualify as fads or movements, but add to the popular confusion when it comes to something as basic as choosing what to eat. There is a lot of talk about the standard American diet (SAD), but the reality is that there is no standard. More than anything, diets in America are substandard, lacking essential nutrients due to soil depletion, unnatural growing conditions, and global toxicity. Instead, Americans are eating too many processed foods loaded with chemicals, simple carbohydrates, and fats designed in laboratories.

Mark, a senior entertainment executive in his late thirties, came to me with a conundrum. He was in good shape externally—a Division 1 athlete in college, he still went to the gym at least three days a week—but he was experiencing significant energy and emotional swings throughout the day, an inability to sleep properly through the night, and bouts of sluggishness, edginess, indigestion, and occasional heartburn. Worse, his recent physical examination had revealed high cholesterol, elevated mercury, and high blood pressure. The disconnect between his high fitness level and low state of well-being confused him. The first question I asked was what he ate. Breakfast was a double espresso with a half packet of sugar. "Not exactly the breakfast of champions," he admitted, but something that fortified him for his stressful work environment. His lunches and dinners were stuck in the college era. They often featured pizza, ice cream, soda, steak and fries, cookies, candy, and burgers.

Though Mark said he needed a change, he was skeptical about cleansing—something he associated with the harsh colon cleanses he'd seen for sale at his vitamin store. I suggested he see it as a business venture: outcome uncertain, but definitely worth the risk. His caffeinated, starchy diet was contributing to his roller-coaster energy and moods. It was full of dairy products, meat, and sugar—all highly acidifying, which contributes to indigestion and heartburn. It was also lacking in key nutrients needed to stay stable, like magnesium, which helps combat stress, or any kind of probiotic food, which would have benefited him in many ways. During the Clean program Mark was required to go without all these things; I was especially interested to see what happened when his sugars and starchy foods got the boot.

When Mark saw me after his third week, he looked great. He'd lost seven pounds as well as an inch from his waistline without losing any athletic strength. But more important, he finally got off the carb-induced roller coaster. "I have more energy, sleep well, and don't crave bad foods or have the ups and downs in mood," he reported, adding that he no longer felt dependent on caffeine. "My brain functions more clearly than at any other point in my life," he reported. To his surprise, his taste buds had reset. "Now that I feel better than I ever have, I just want to eat better." The skeptic had turned convert to an existence free of junk food and Starbucks.

The problem of not knowing what to eat is older than any theory ever invented to correct it. It started when humans began thinking about food. Animals in the wild don't think about what they will have for lunch; eating happens. Humans lost touch with their instincts, and now we have to study thick books before we can safely prepare a meal. The only one I trust for such an important decision is the book of nature. When animals live in their natural environments, the way nature designed, they do not get sick. But even if observing nature will not tell us exactly what we humans should be eating by natural design, it becomes clear that whatever we are doing is not it. Animals eat plants, seeds, nuts, and each other, always raw. No animal always eats three times a day. No other animal eats every other living species on the planet. No wild animal eats for fun or out of sadness. No other mammals continue to drink milk after they stop breastfeeding. No animal in the wild is obese, and diseases are rare, mostly a result of exposure to our chemical poisoning of the planet.

There are many other questions that will help you get a more complete picture of the present dilemma when feeding our families and ourselves.

How much and how often should we eat? With the thought, "If it's good for us, having access to it all the time will make us happier," we began to surround ourselves with food and make sure our bellies had something in them for most of the day. We figured out ways to grow crops cheaply in mass quantity. We take three meals a day for granted, but it is no more than a social construct (as you will read in a later chapter). Eating constantly without resting the digestive system may be at the root of our inability to detoxify naturally.

Where do we buy our food? The best possible source of foods is the local farmers' market. They sell foods that are in season, which is the way that animals eat in the wild. Buying organic foods at the supermarket would be the next choice. There is some confusion with the labeling, so it can be tricky, since the word "organic" still means different things. But if you buy truly organic food, you avoid many of the toxic chemicals described above. At my corner deli in New York, it is February and I find watermelon from Mexico, blueberries from Chile, apples from Colombia, bananas from Venezuela, and oranges from California. These were transported thousands of miles over many days. To keep these fruits from spoiling in transit, farmers had to pick them before they were ripe, before they had stocked up their nutrient reserves. This contributes to the depletion of nutrients in our diets.

What food did our food eat? The problem of nutrient depletion starts at the beginning of the food chain. Plants are grown in soils that are depleted of minerals. Mass production of food leads to abuse of the land, and fertilizers do not deliver their promise. Vital foods, such as vegetables and fruits, are rendered nutritionally inert, because they are deficient in trace minerals that used to be abundant in rich, healthy soils. (Soil degradation is one of Earth's silent crises—it is only now beginning to get attention, but it is slowly harming the whole planet's food-cultivating ability.) The Vitamin A in tomatoes has gone down 43 percent in the last six decades; the Vitamin C in potatoes has decreased 57 percent. Unless you bought your vegetables and fruits at a farmers' market, they have most likely been harvested long before ripeness (depleting them of essential nutrients your cells need to do their chemistry), and unless you know otherwise, your produce almost definitely came from nutrient-depleted soils.

As you will read in a later chapter, the process of detoxification is significantly diminished when the nutrients needed for its chemical reactions are not available. The most popular fertilizer, NPK, provides only three (sodium, phosphorus, potassium) of the fifty-plus minerals needed for healthy plants. Therefore, plants from soil using NPK alone will develop weak immune systems. When irritated by insects or chemicals, such as insecticides, plants develop an inflammatory reaction, increasing the content of omega-6 fatty acids, a pro-inflammatory nutrient, and decreasing the production of omega-3, a potent anti-inflammatory nutrient. When animals are fed in an unnatural way, they tend to get sick. Farmed fish have less fish oil (omega-3 fatty acids). Corn-fed cows develop gastritis, inflammation, and infections and need antibiotics. When we eat these plants, fish, and cows, we are eating inflammation, which, among other things, makes us more prone to coronary artery disease (the blockages in the arteries leading to heart attacks), cancer, and other chronic diseases.

Who on this planet lives longer, healthier lives? There are a few communities in which people's life expectancy is much higher than that of the rest of the world's population. Their inhabitants not only live longer, but their lives are also more active, productive, and, ultimately, more fulfilling. The areas where they live are called blue zones. There is one in the south of Ecuador, one on the islands south of Italy, and one in the desert in southern California. When these and a few other blue zones were visited and observed, the people all shared similar habits. These habits were simple. They grew everything they ate using only compost, water, and sun (no chemicals). Food was predominantly plants, mostly raw and always seasonal. Their animals were fed and raised in natural ways. They took longer to prepare or cook their food, a process more like a ritual than a chore. They chewed their food ten times longer than we do on average. They spent time in the sun. They moved a lot. They also enjoyed rich foods and wine—occasionally. All of them had strong family bonds and treasured friendships. Meals were eaten sitting at a table with family and friends. Life was lived with a strong sense of purpose and belonging to the community.

One cannot argue with success. As a doctor, when I answer the frequently asked question of what to eat for a long, healthy life, my patients who follow my advice start eating like the people who live in the blue zones. What I prescribe is geared toward creating the conditions by which the digestive system is put to relative rest, so the detoxification system can wake from its relative hibernating state and the organs and systems involved in the process of cleaning our insides can have everything they need, when they need it, to complete their job. This is what Clean is about.

CHAPTER FIVE

How Toxins Affect Your Health

Each toxic molecule creates a cascade of reactions that expands like the radiating ripples around a single drop of water on the surface of a calm lake. You can follow the ripples as far as your eye can see. In the same way, you can follow the chemical footprint of each toxin long after the toxin itself initiated the chain of events. But a tropical storm on that same lake is a very different picture. Millions of individual drops, each starting a ripple that collides with other ripples, make it impossible for an observer to distinguish one ripple from another. In fact, when the storm gets real intense, there are no more ripples. It just becomes a new kind of general surface pattern.

THE DROP

Toxins have many ways of interfering with the normal physiology of life. They can do it in a very unique and specific way, like arsenic, a deadly poison that causes asphyxia by blocking the usage of oxygen needed for the full metabolism of glucose. Toxins may block an enzyme needed for an important body function. Or they may stimulate a specific body function in such persistent ways that it begins to cause damage. Caffeine, when consumed many times a day, stimulates the adrenal glands, resulting in a fight-or-flight response, in which the body prepares for intense action by increasing heart rate, blood pressure, alertness, and temperature. When caffeine is taken in persistently over a period of time, one can exhaust the adrenal system and not even realize caffeine was the cause. In fact, when started on the Clean program and asked to stop caffeine completely, many patients complain because they think they can only function if they have their coffee. Other toxins kill the good bacteria in the intestinal tract, block oxygen from binding to red blood cells, interfere with DNA synthesis by switching genes on and off, or block the absorption of different vitamins.

Molecules that carry an electric charge cause irritation and damage by facilitating oxidation, the much talked about "oxidants." The process is similar to what happens to metals when they rust. These toxins are neutralized by anti-oxidants, abundant in raw vegetables and fruits. There are also toxins that interfere with the absorption of necessary nutrients, such as the prescription medications listed in appendix "Prescription Drugs and Nutritional Depletion."

Mercury, a toxic metal, is known as the "great mimicker." Mercury toxicity can present as almost any other disease. Toxic levels of this metal can trigger a chain of reactions that end up causing psychiatric imbalances, cancer, autoimmune diseases, or anemia, to name a few.

Each of the examples above describes how one type of toxic molecule interferes with our ability to maintain the balance necessary for a healthy life. We can describe the individual mechanism for any of the many of the toxins mentioned so far in the book. It is even possible that scientists could one day understand how each of them alters our chemistry. But what is certainly impossible is to ever understand in detail how they interact when many of them are present together in the same organism.

Overexposure to Heavy Metals

For the last eight years, thirty-eight-year-old Sara has been experiencing joint pains, most severely in her lower back and hips. She has gone to many doctors and specialists. She was found to have antibodies against her own cells' nuclei, a subtype called anti-Ro. Though her specialist could not tell her why this happened, he gave her a diagnosis of ankylosing spondylitis, a form of autoimmune arthritis. Painkillers, anti-inflammatories, and steroid injections to manage the pain became a part of her life. Finally, a course of chemotherapy was recommended to inactivate the confused immune system of her own body. Her own "natural instinct" rejected the idea, and she came to me for help on the recommendation of a friend.

One question puzzled her. I asked if she had silver amalgam fillings in her mouth. She did. My questions also revealed she ate sushi a lot, which is known to have a high heavy-metal content. I asked her to do a twenty-four-hour urine challenge test with DMSA and found she had toxic levels of mercury and arsenic. We don't know why one person is more susceptible than another—but clearly she needed to correct this. Although I didn't tell her to stop the chemotherapy, I asked if she would put it on pause for a few months, since she'd already had eight years of pain and a different approach was merited. She agreed.

Sara completed three weeks of the Clean program and afterwards started oral chelation, a process using a chemical agent called DMSA to bind to heavy metals and draw them out. (This is a long-term treatment; it must be done with professional supervision and on a schedule to ensure the reintroduction of beneficial minerals, which are also drawn out in the process.) Midway through, her grayish skin tone turned to pink, and her joint pain started to lessen. Her optimism returned, and she simply felt and looked healthier. At the time of this writing, we are still waiting to find out if, after the completion of her heavy-metal detox, she will show a reversal of the antibody production.

If you suffer from a chronic disease that puzzles your primary-care doctor, does not respond to any treatment for too long, or responds, but immediately another set of symptoms takes their place, find a healthcare practitioner who is trained in Functional Medicine to help you get the right test. Mercury or any of the other toxic metals could be a daily visitor in your life without your even knowing it. See the chart of possible sources of toxic metals in Appendix "Unexpected Common Sources of Heavy-Metal Exposure."

THE STORM

In my practice, I needed to find a way to think about toxicity that allowed me to help my patients. Looking at every individual toxin and trying to isolate its chemical ripples from the others was too confusing. Once again, when I took a step back from the detailed level of individual molecules to the perspective of the whole person, a much clearer picture started to emerge. The storm of toxins on the lake of the human body started to create patterns similar to symptoms and diseases I knew too well.

Puffiness

When Ari came to see me, he described some of the side effects of eight years of married life and having small children in the house. His fridge had had a makeover for the worse. Diet Cokes, cupcakes, and chocolates were there to tempt him, and with more than a few bites here and there his belly was getting a makeover too. He told me, almost laughing, "For the first time I'm feeling like a tired old person—and no one looks at me on the beach anymore." Though he was resistant to the idea of replacing two meals a day with liquids, he successfully completed the Clean program. Several pounds came off over the first two weeks. By the third week he reported something surprising. Not only had the extra eleven pounds he'd been carrying for years slipped off his frame, but his skin looked tighter and firmer. "As I was shaving, I realized the face in the mirror looking back at me was different. It looked ten years younger," he said.

Most Eastern forms of medicine talk about mucus as toxic waste in our body. It is a very different understanding than we have here, which has mostly to do with runny noses. When I first heard a doctor of Chinese medicine talk about mucus being present in the entire system, it sounded laughable to me. I remember thinking, "What is he talking about?" So I asked him, "Where is this 'mucus'?" Dr. William So, a Korean acupuncturist from a multigenerational family of healers who has since taught me a tremendous amount about Chinese medicine, replied calmly, "Everywhere. It's in the cells, around the cells, in your blood, in your guts. It's even in your thoughts."

India's Ayurvedic tradition calls this heavy, toxic substance that accumulates in the body *amma* and doesn't distinguish whether the source is physical or mental. It says that all stressors on the system, from toxic foods to toxic thoughts, manifest as a mucusy heaviness in the body, which is the first stage of disease. When you are trained to see it, you can detect its presence right away. The clinical sign of it is what I call "puffiness." It's a symptom that Western medicine doesn't even have a name for and is largely overlooked, even when we're staring right at it. (This is one of the limitations of the Western model of medicine: if a condition doesn't have a name, doctors don't even see it.)

But just look around, and it's evident that almost everybody living a modern life is "puffed up" to some extent:

- The skin might be a little saggy, instead of being taut and firm. There may be dark circles under the eyes on waking up.

- There is bloating around the body, and sometimes there are extra pounds that won't budge, even if the person counts calories and exercises. Clothes feel tighter, or the belly is puffed, even on a thin person. Often there's a turgid state especially in the bowels; movement gets stuck and constipation results.

- In the morning, the tongue might have a white film on the back part of it. If it's there, it should be scraped off with a tongue scraper. (A significant amount may indicate that you have been eating and drinking late at night when the digestive system should be resting.)

- There may be a heaviness or torpor in the system, which is sometimes also felt as a lack of clarity or joy.

Even people who consider themselves healthy and fit are familiar with this puffy state—maybe on some days more than others, depending on how well they've been eating and drinking.

Mucus is a natural defense response against irritation. If you inhale some cayenne pepper while cooking, your nose runs because it's trying to get that irritant out. The mucus is the gel that first surrounds the pepper particle so it can't burn the sensitive nose lining and then facilitates sliding the irritant out.

Too much of the wrong food or other toxins from the environment cause irritation also. But this time it's inside, where you don't see or feel it happening. The toxins irritate the sensitive wall of the intestines. When the cells there get irritated, just like in the nose, they defend themselves by creating a protective buffer of sticky mucus to separate themselves from the toxic particles. This can be the beginning of a constipated state, something that is typically made worse by the degraded state of the intestinal flora.

Next, the irritants slip through the lining of the intestines and into the blood vessels on the other side, irritating them as well. As the toxins are carried around in the bloodstream, they trigger irritation everywhere they go, which generates mucus in and around the cells of the muscles and tissues. This mucus is acidic, so it adds to the already overly acidified state of the body. And because it's like a sponge, sucking up water, mucus swells the cells and "puffs you up"—you look and feel bloated and dulled.

When your nose makes mucus, it comes out easily. You blow your nose to help it move and then it's gone. When mucus is being made deeper inside the body, it gets stuck. Of course, there is a pathway for it to get out—the mucus needs to be pulled back out of the cells, carried back in the blood to the intestinal wall, and then moved back across the wall into the lumen, where it can get eliminated. But this requires resources, and if the volume of inbound toxins is high, the body's economy of energy is tilted toward containing the attack. It is so busy surrounding the irritants that it can't get to the job of carrying them out. It's as if all the garbage handlers in the city are bagging the trash and none of them are left to drive it to the dump. Add to this the fact that digestion and the metabolism of food also take energy, and there's little left for full detoxification. The more we eat and snack, the less energy is left over for throwing out the trash. The mucus builds up and doesn't leave. Stubborn weight lingers on the body, the puffiness in the face won't go down even after a diet, and things don't change until a concentrated period of detoxification starts.

Fortunately, the opposite also proves true. When you eat sparingly, take in nutrients that promote detoxification, and start exercising, you "de-puff." You may experience this after a few days of cutting out bad foods on your own. After several days on an effective detoxification program or cleanse, the effects are much deeper. As mucus is released from its sites all around the body, toxins are stripped of their mucus coating and make their way back into bloodstream for eventual neutralization and elimination. In a kind of natural "shedding," excess weight caused by the water and mucus begins to melt away. Often, as with Ari, the person loses some significant extra pounds of weight—the body self-corrects. Eyes get much whiter and brighter, and skin firms up so much that women patients often say their friends ask if they got a facelift.

Not surprisingly, a sense of clarity and lightness return to body and mind after a cleanse. Western medicine has historically separated body and mind, but Eastern medicine never has divided them. They are two aspects of the whole. *Amma* therefore refers to both the congesting mucus created by toxicity and

The Face: The First Clue

Your face is the part of you that you probably look at most. It's also where signs of toxicity are most evident if you know how to spot them. Taut skin that pops back into place immediately when you pull it is healthy; the less elastic it is, the more "puffy" or mucusy you are. The sagging of skin that we consider a "normal, natural" sign of aging isn't necessarily so. Many elders in communities that eat clean, traditional diets have taut skin, uplifted around the bone structure, until the end of their lives. Pimples and dark circles under the eyes are also a clue to toxic buildup. Look at your skin with a magnifying mirror. Can you see pores all over? If you see little depressions in the surface, like the skin of an orange, there is mucus and water accumulation in the skin, which has caused the areas around the pores to swell or puff up, making the pores more pronounced.

the heavy, dulled thoughts and emotions that keep you "stuck" in a negative mind-set. Both are considered to have a dense nature and therefore to attract each other. Vital, fresh foods and inspired, uplifting thoughts also attract each other and go together. Too many negative emotions or thoughts will make you crave the foods that end up generating the production of mucus and will cause you to fall into lazy lifestyle patterns (like not exercising) that help it accumulate. Similarly, it can happen the other way around: the formation of excess mucus from poor foods, irritation, and stagnancy in the body makes the appearance of negative emotions and thoughts much more likely. It's another way of saying, "We eat what we are."

Constipation

Annabelle, a tall, slender twenty-six-year-old, had an enviably healthy lifestyle. She rarely ate any kind of processed foods; she prepared mostly organic, fresh meals at home. She exercised and didn't drink or smoke. To her friends she was the poster child for health. But, unknown to them, she had an ongoing battle with her bowels. For years, regular bowel movements were elusive. She used caffeine, herbal laxatives, and sometimes over-the-counter laxatives to try to stimulate elimination. The condition upset her. She felt bloated much of the time and psychologically it was taking far too much of her energy and attention.

During her first Clean program, she removed the primary irritating foods, got on a schedule of not eating after dinner, and built up her intestinal flora. The first two weeks were hard; she still got constipated until she started taking a strong herbal laxative. She also got a few colonic treatments. The third week, her body began to kick into action. Relieved of certain foods and caffeine and given some time to restore itself, her bowel function was finding its way back to normal. With astonishment Annabelle reported that her daily bowel movements were in excess of anything she'd had before, especially toward the end of the program. I told her that she was shedding some of the toxicity held throughout her body, in her cells and tissues. Her energy levels increased, and she experienced great clarity.

After Clean, she reported a different relationship to food; she had a new hunger and enjoyed eating, because meals were no longer something guaranteed to slow her down. Yet her newly improved condition required some maintenance. On adding back ingredients from her old diet, like cheese or pasta, her elimination slowed down again. Annabelle had to learn her triggers and keep a Clean diet for her bowels to work their best.

Constipation is one of the most frequent health complaints in the Western world. Laxatives are big business in the United States, and many people spend a lot of effort, time, and money trying to manage this symptom. Some try natural methods and small dietary changes, like adding more fruit, which may or may not improve the situation. But until they repair and restore intestinal integrity and remove certain foods for good, the solutions are often ineffective. (For example, excessive fruit can actually add to the sugar that feeds dysbiosis, the presence of yeast or of harmful intestinal bacteria.) The situation is much worse than we acknowledge, because what most people consider a "normal" state of bowel elimination is actually constipation in the picture of total wellness. An elimination after each meal is closer to what is natural for the body—but it's not the common experience today.

Not all mucus is bad. There is a thin film of beneficial mucus on the intestinal wall. It is where the intestinal flora lives, it has antimicrobial properties for bad bacteria. But eating too many carbohydrates and dairy products, which are all hard to digest, promotes the formation of a stickier mucus that buffers irritation. This denser mucus partially blocks food absorption while slowing the bowels. When partially digested food sits in the intestines, yeast and bad bacteria have more time to devour more food. They flourish and emit more of their toxic waste, which numbs nerves and weakens muscle, causing further stagnancy in the colon and therefore delay in the release of feces. When stools sit inside the colon too long, their toxins may get reabsorbed back into the body, which may be experienced as the headaches and body pain that can accompany constipation. If this is a regular state, the constipation becomes chronic, partly because the good bacteria die off as the bad ones flourish—and good bacteria go together with regular bowel movements.

For a detox program to be complete, it must help to correct constipation by eliminating the irritating toxins that cause mucus buildup. Different people are affected differently, but the most common mucus-forming foods are wheat, dairy products, refined sugars, and excessive red meat. A complete detox also replenishes the good bacteria while killing the bad. And it begins the process of restoring some of the nutrients essential for a healthy bowel, for example, iodine, necessary for proper thyroid function and therefore beneficial for the bowels, and magnesium, needed for the muscular contraction of the bowels. The Clean program is complete, since it replenishes nutrients, eliminates toxin exposure, and enhances the neutralization and elimination of damaging molecules and the mucus that was formed to buffer their irritation. Its benefits go deep.

Calming the mind through a daily meditation practice can also have significant benefits on this state. If anger, greed, and other negative emotions are the initial cause of constipation, as older traditions of healing and well-being say, then we need to look beyond the physical realm for clues to this ongoing condition. Off-loading the toxins of stress that congest the body is as important as taking in correct foods. We rarely make the time to disempower the toxic thoughts in our minds as our ancestors did with practices of meditation and contemplation—perhaps if we did, laxatives would not be such top-selling items at the drugstore. Sometimes the root of the problem is not something that can be solved by supplements and diet alone.

There are so many connections between nutrition and intestinal health that it is almost impossible to say in an exact, mathematical way what each person will need. Covering all the possible needs without overloading is the hallmark of a sound detox program like Clean.

Allergies

Tony, a businessman, was in good control of his health. He practiced yoga and exercised regularly, ate at good restaurants when he went out, and cooked with high-quality organic ingredients. But in the three years since turning forty, he'd noticed a dip in his energy. He was getting more headaches than in his younger days. His body wasn't as lean as he'd expected from all his yoga; he had love handles that wouldn't leave. The most pronounced change was seasonal allergies that got worse each year. They were now so bad he had to take prescription medication. He had heard that allergies were getting worse in today's "dirtier" environment. He hoped a detox might help his problem and get him off the medication.

On questioning Tony more closely about his lifestyle, I found out that he ate bread and pasta frequently and loved ice cream. I explained that his diet, more than the dirty environment he lived in, was probably the primary cause of his problem. Wheat is a classic trigger of allergic responses. So are dairy products and refined sugars. They irritate and erode the intestinal walls, resulting in a "leaky gut," the origin of inadequate allergic responses. Intestinal dysbiosis also contributes to exaggerated allergic responses. I suggested he follow an elimination diet for a couple of weeks, cutting out those sweet, milky foods along with the wheat, which would allow any leaks in the intestinal wall to heal. Then I recommended a three-week cleanse to restore a healthy intestinal environment by repopulating it with good bacteria.

Tony followed the instructions with the dedication of a true yogi, though his first week without ice cream he said was horrible. After three weeks he reported with some shock that he'd lost twenty-two pounds. He simply did not understand where those pounds had come from, as he had never considered himself overweight. He was leaner, though not overly thin, with the same good muscle tone and shape from his yoga. His love handles had almost entirely disappeared, and his skin was taut and firm. He also reported having the energy he'd had at age twenty. But the most important change revealed itself over the year that followed. He did not have seasonal allergies at all. Removing the root cause of the allergy, the damaged intestinal wall that keeps the gut-associated lymphatic tissue (GALT) overstimulated, had allowed for true healing to happen. Not only had the accumulated mucus been removed; his intestinal wall had started to heal.

Allergies are one of the most common symptoms of toxicity. But detecting the cause isn't as easy as staying away from the things that make you sneeze. Allergic responses to food don't necessarily play out in an obvious cause-and-effect way, like drinking milk and immediately getting hives or a stomach cramp. They can be delayed by hours, expressing themselves as diarrhea or headaches later in the day. Or sometimes the thing that seems to trigger the attack is only the "straw that broke the camel's back," as it was for Tony. The true cause of his problem was the irritating foods and toxic chemicals that caused a leaky gut and kept his immune system on heightened alert mode throughout the year, not simply the pollen he breathed in at the change of seasons, which tipped his system into crisis. A cursory look at the problem of allergies often leads to an incorrectly identified source. Trying to avoid trees and plants would not have cured Tony—likely some other trigger would have become the instigator of itchy eyes and nose.

As Tony learned, if the intestinal wall is intact and the good flora alive, the gut-associated lymphatic tissue is awake, but calm. If the intestinal wall is damaged, it is hyperactive and ready to cause havoc, even when the allergen makes contact with the interior of the body at a far-off point, like pollen inhaled in through the airway. The body picks up the message that invaders have arrived and initiates a defense response, forming mucus and calling your attention through itchiness. Removing the most common irritating foods from the diet during the Clean program is the first step to restoring order in the body and preventing allergies. But because ice cream, wheat, or whatever food item is the true cause of the problem seems unconnected to the sneezing, eliminating foods from the diet is not always the obvious step to take. Years go by and we are still eating irritating foods while suffering symptoms that we are convinced are triggered by anything but food.

Each of us has our own constitutional weakness that is affected by a problem in the intestines. Tony didn't have any symptoms of constipation or bloating, yet his damaged intestinal environment manifested in the area of his weakness—nasal and bronchial irritation. Others might be doubled over with belly cramps from excess gas, while still others experience the downward dip of exhaustion or foggy brain.

Depression

Thirty-year-old Kate had been feeling increasingly depressed. She had consulted a psychiatrist who told her (in an echo of my own case) that she had a "chemical imbalance." She was prescribed an antidepressant and when small doses didn't help her mood, her prescription was increased to the maximum dose. This high dose bothered Kate, who mentioned she felt uncomfortable taking medication for her sadness at all—but at least the pain in her heart and the anxiety that made breathing difficult at times had subsided. It was a secondary, but equally upsetting problem that had brought her to me. She had gained twenty-five pounds while on the medication, and the shame about that was starting to be as painful as the sadness that the antidepressant had improved.

I told Kate that her antidepressant is part of a group of drugs called selective serotonin reuptake inhibitors (SSRIs). They are designed to help with low serotonin levels—not by increasing the amount produced, but by letting the amounts available in the body stick around longer before being inactivated. Although they can be very beneficial in cases of moderate depression to kick-start someone to a more stable place, they can sometimes mask the real problem: something in the factory of the intestines, where the majority of the serotonin is produced, has gone awry.

Instead of relying forever on an outside source for something Kate was designed by nature to make in her own body, we wanted to correct whatever was causing her to underproduce the neurotransmitter. In addition, I told her that one of the most common issues I see among women her age is a sluggish thyroid gland, due to mental stress, allergies, and inadequate nutrition. This influences both weight gain and depression. By giving her body a recharge and a "reset" through a cleanse, the inner serotonin production gets a chance to improve and the thyroid can bounce back into full action, helping to regulate weight again. Kate ended up doing six weeks of Clean, because she was feeling so great that she didn't want to change anything.

In total she lost thirty pounds and looked better than ever. I worked in conjunction with her psychiatrist to slowly taper her off the antidepressant.

When your intestinal environment is damaged and inflamed, there is a slow reduction of natural serotonin levels, because so much of your serotonin is made in the intestines under the right conditions. When this happens, it physically changes the way you are getting signals about what to feel and how to respond to the world. Your experiences of moods and feelings will change for the worse, shifting to apathy, a dulled anesthetized state, or serious lows. This explanation could be seen as a modern scientific understanding of *amma*'s torpor of the spirit. Both are caused by toxicity.

As anyone with a more complex understanding of the psyche and physiology knows, the picture of depression is far more intricate than this. For one thing, many other neurotransmitters are involved that may also be out of balance, whether from a lack of nutrients or subtler imbalances in other parts of the body. Then add to this the toxins from the problems of the heart and soul that evade a physical examination, and it is impossible to say that there is ever a single cause of depression. I would never have presumed to tell Kate

Manufacturing Happiness

Serotonin production is greatly influenced by diet. Like everything in the body, serotonin is built from the nutrients we obtain from food. It uses certain amino acids as building blocks, especially the one known as tryptophan, which comes from high-protein foods. Levels of tryptophan have hugely declined in the modern diet. When we ate wild animals that foraged on grasses and other plants, we got more tryptophan in our diets. Grain-fed animals have much less of it, just as they have less omega-3 fatty acids. In addition, the natural production of serotonin is inhibited by caffeine, alcohol, and aspartame; a lack of sunlight; and a lack of exercise. After repairing the damaged intestinal environment, creating a Wellness Plan with a nutrient-balanced diet and possibly a regime of supplements that include probiotics (foods supplying beneficial intestinal bacteria) is an important step in sustaining more stable serotonin levels.

whether the root of her suffering started in the body (that low neurotransmitter production was causing her low spirits) or in the spirit (that her spirit was generating a physical symptom to get her attention).

But serotonin levels are something we can optimize just in case and work with that. Time and time again, I've witnessed how restoring intestinal integrity reactivates the major serotonin factory in the intestines and causes the mental fog, sadness, or distress to melt away. This can be the massive first step toward real healing of the spirit. Frequently, as Kate experienced, the patient who is already on an antidepressant is able to reduce the dosage and often stop taking it entirely. (This should always be done under the care of the prescribing physician and never on your own.)

Antidepressants, when used conscientiously, can serve an important purpose. In cases of moderate or severe depression they can be the "bridge" that helps patients shift from a place where they are floundering to a place where they feel some solid ground. Like any drug, they need to be neutralized and eliminated by the liver, so they add to the toxic load. But antidepressants can be a good tool to use while repairing the intestinal flora during and after a detox program. Since the brain is "plastic," meaning it is always changing and modifying, antidepressants can help create some new neural pathways through which your experience of the world gets processed. You are creating a new and improved memory of what it's like to feel better over the few months it might take to restore your intestinal flora and get your intestines to manufacture their own serotonin, reestablishing the pathways to a happier perception of the world.

Because most antidepressants only work for a while and many people build up a tolerance after six months to a year, to treat depression without restoring the conditions in the body is negligent. Often patients are simply put on higher doses or on a second or third antidepressant. To rely on antidepressants as the only course of action long-term is like whipping a weak horse to make it run. It may run, but it will collapse after a while. Meanwhile the side effects of the medications—from decreased libido, impotence, insomnia, and weight gain or loss to dry mouth and more—can accumulate. (The most tragic side effect of all is suicide, which is little discussed in the medical world.) When, however, patients increase their serotonin naturally, it's as if we brought a hundred new horses into the race and let the weak one go out to pasture and enjoy the grass.

Irritable Bowel Syndrome

An estimated 10 to 15 percent of Americans have irritable bowel syndrome; it accounts for 12 percent of primary-care visits. The word "syndrome" can include all sorts of symptoms, including bloating and digestive pain, but classically IBS refers to a situation where the bowels have extreme reactions with no predictability—such as alternating between constipation and diarrhea—and seemingly acting with a mind of their own. This phrase is apt. IBS is actually a kind of "depression of the intestines," linked to diminished amounts of serotonin just like psychological depression. The nerve cells in the intestines orchestrate digestion and cause the muscle of the intestines to contract. When serotonin levels are inappropriate, the intestine gets disturbed, causing the alternating bouts of too much or too little activity or general discomfort. These symptoms are also exacerbated by chronic constipation. When toxic waste sits in the colon, the intelligent nervous system of the intestine can alternate between primal panic, giving you diarrhea to get rid of the toxins, and paralysis, making you bloated.

The concept of healing IBS naturally by restoring serotonin production and removing toxicity is not widely discussed. This is ironic, given that modern medicine pioneered the idea of treating IBS patients with antidepressants. The protocol evolved accidentally, after enough patients with depression who were being treated with SSRIs were unexpectedly getting relief from IBS (not surprising, given what we know about neurotransmitters and the scope of the suffering, which can in the most extreme cases lead to a high rate of unnecessary surgeries such as cholecystectomies, hysterectomies, appendectomies, and back surgeries). The medication these patients were given for their "psychological" symptoms alleviated the bowel conditions so well that this treatment has now become standard protocol for IBS, whether the patient is depressed or not. Yet little discussion has gone into *why* the SSRIs are actually helping the patients' IBS to improve.

DIAGNOSING TOXICITY

How do you even know if toxicity is affecting you? The symptoms are different from person to person, but when you are trained to see them, the clues are consistent. I always take a good look at my patients through my detox glasses.

Remember Tony's tiredness and allergies? Kate's depression and weight gain? Robert, in his sixties, suffers from unpredictable bowels, which only adds more stress to his high-pressure job. Told he has IBS, he assumes it's something he has to live with and is not something he can fix on his own.

Tony's, Kate's, and Robert's symptoms are common among my busy, hardworking patients. So are skin and sinus problems, fatigue and bloating after eating, constipation, headaches, muscle or joint pain, and arthritis-like tendencies as well as a general low-grade state of emotional malaise.

Their different responses show why, in general, doctors and patients today are detox-blind. How would we know that a single protocol of reversing the toxic state could relieve many of their problems, when the problems are all so different? The body's response to toxicity is a complex web of possible reactions, not a single reaction that looks or feels the same in everyone.

On one level, toxicity goes hand in hand with the buildup of something that Eastern traditions call *amma* and that we simply call "mucus." It is responsible for the puffed-up, bloated, heavy, or dulled feeling in body and mind that is so common today. At the next level, the toxic irritation goes deeper, causing allergic reactions to everyday things. And on yet another level, it stimulates the body's immune system to get hyperactive and make mistakes in what it's fighting; it starts attacking the body's own cells and tissues, causing autoimmune disorders from gluten intolerance to arthritis and others.

What's the consistent story behind the different cases? All these symptoms of dysfunction have as their root cause a state of irritation and mucus formation. And all of them begin to get cleared up when we remove the conditions that cause the irritation and facilitate the elimination of mucus.

GLOBAL INNER CLIMATE CHANGES: THE WEATHER ON TOXICITY TV

Our bodies are a wonder. Consider the trillions of chemical reactions that happen instant after instant, the sum total of which adds up to our experience of life. It is impossible to affect a single one of those chemical reactions without affecting many others. Yet modern medicine has evolved in the other direction, away from seeing these balancing agents as a single, connected picture. Western medicine came to value superspecialists over generalists. One doctor looks at and understands mostly throats; another, the lungs; a different one looks at your heart; and so on. We need to shift our attention to the whole picture and create the conditions for the most apparently insignificant chemical reactions to happen as they should. The Clean program does just that. I think of it as molecular acupuncture, a comparison from the mind of Jeffrey Bland, the father of Functional Medicine: a small action in one place, like restoring the right balance of pro- to anti-inflammatory fats or shifting the body's acid-base ratio, triggers a cascade of positive effects in the whole body.

When a butterfly flaps its wings in Japan, the chain of cause and effect may well end up manifesting as a tornado in Argentina. In the same way, a failed chemical reaction involving a few molecules in your liver might just show up as a tumor in your brain. Everything is connected. One little point in space and time may trigger a cascade of reactions that affect a much larger system downstream—one on whose delicate balance life depends.

The reason many of these problems persist and get worse with time is that modern medicine tends to focus on making a diagnosis, instead of looking at what is behind it. What is the diagnosis behind all other diagnoses?

Many years ago, we started noticing that environmental disasters were on the rise: storms, hurricanes, floods, wildfires, melting of the ice caps. Early on, they seemed isolated, unrelated accidents of nature. Slowly the dots were connected. All these disasters were related and had something in common: global warming.

Inside our bodies, a similar crisis is brewing. The massive load of toxins we are exposed to changes our inner climate the way greenhouse gases change Earth's atmosphere.

Acid Rain

Just like in an aquarium or a freshwater lake, where the degree of acidity must be carefully maintained for fish to survive, the environment inside our arteries needs to stay in a certain acid-base range or the cells circulating inside will die. The waste products of normal metabolism are almost exclusively acids, so the body is constantly neutralizing acids as part of daily life. Nature is the main provider of balancing alkaline molecules, in foods like green leafy vegetables. But modern "staple foods" like sugar, dairy products, meat, coffee, and junk food are acidifying. So are medications. So is stress, because the higher metabolic rates and adrenalin and cortisol created during stress speed up acidifying processes. (This is why practices like meditation help control excess acid formation.) It's not an understatement to say that modern life is an acid-forming process.

Overly acidic conditions slowly but surely corrode our inner terrain to the point of causing damage. Acidity may corrode arteries, resulting in heart attacks or strokes. It may corrode joints, resulting in arthritis. It certainly promotes the malfunctioning of key processes like oxygen exchange in the red blood cells, inflammation, blood clotting, hormone production, and nerve cell conduction. In fact, I can't think of one single chemical reaction in the body that is not affected by acidity. You will be reducing acidity during Clean by removing the foods that are acidifying, lowering stress, and boosting detoxification.

Drought

The modern-day phenomenon of nutritional deficiency is devastating to our health. Everything that happens in the body does so through chemical reactions. Digestion, healing, and communicating between cells all take place through little acts of chemistry; these chemical reactions need a certain supply of naturally occurring ingredients. We are designed to get most of these micronutrients from foods. If they are missing, the chemical reactions simply don't happen, imbalances start, and over time sickness and disease develop. Many people have heard they need to supplement their diet with omega-3 fatty acids (fish oils); it's popular knowledge. But there are three newly identified deficiencies that are about to become just as popular.

MAGNESIUM

Magnesium, a mineral, stabilizes and calms the nervous system and relaxes muscles. It is hard to absorb to begin with (only 10 percent of the magnesium ingested is absorbed), but its depletion is one of the contributing factors to the modern epidemic of stress, anxiety, high blood pressure, depression, edema, memory loss, irritability, and weakness.

VITAMIN D

Vitamin D is integrally involved in a multitude of vital processes. It helps the deposition of calcium in the bones and regulates the immune system, so a lack of it will contribute to bone disease and cause a predisposition to frequent infections. It plays an important role in mood chemistry and is critical for heart health. Because this vitamin needs sunlight for activation and we have shielded ourselves from the sunlight by living inside buildings, traveling in cars, and covering every inch of skin with clothing and sun protection creams, there is a new worldwide epidemic of vitamin D deficiency. Expect more diseases to be linked to the lack of this wonder vitamin soon.

IODINE

Iodine is the latest deficiency to come to my awareness at the time of this writing. It is the main building block for the production of thyroid hormones, which are responsible for keeping the furnace of our metabolism going.

Saving Millions to Own a Penny

Chronic undernourishment contributes, ironically, to one of the other crises of our time, overeating and obesity. When the body is starving for a certain trace mineral it needs, it will disrupt the normal signals that tell you to stop eating so that you consume more food in the hopes of grabbing the missing nutrient. All the extra food consumed has to go somewhere—and is typically stored as fat. If the diet is deficient in zinc, for example, which is common today, the body won't give a "satisfied" signal until it's found what it needs, even if that means eating three pounds of food to get a microgram of zinc. Doctors sometimes report a curious syndrome in which people with an iron deficiency get an urge to eat paint, because their bodies are desperate for metal. This very unnatural act is highly toxic—it causes lead poisoning.

Without sufficient amounts, weight gain becomes an issue. This is only one of the consequences of deficient thyroid production due to iodine deficiency (but a critical one, as obesity is becoming a major problem now affecting millions of children). Modern science is now linking it to many other diseases like cancer, heart disease, and depression. It is implicated in the wave of thyroid depletion I see especially among women today, a problem that that my colleague Dr. Frank Lipman brilliantly diagnoses and treats as one of the components of an invisible syndrome in modern medicine that he calls "Spent," described in chapter 7.

The process of detoxification depends on chemicals that our body used to obtain from a balanced diet of nutrient-filled foods. The liver is where the bulk of the detox chemistry happens, and it requires a whole shopping list of natural ingredients, such as vitamins and minerals found in natural, whole foods as well as a good stock of antioxidants. It is like having a well-stocked cleaning supply cupboard, so you can clean your house efficiently and well. But because of nutritional deficiency, your liver struggles, unable to fulfill its function of detoxification. The Clean program restores your supplies by adding specific nutrients to your diet that may have been missing. In addition, it addresses the lack of antioxidants in the standard American diet.

Seventy percent of Earth's surface is water; our bodies are also seventy percent water. It is one of the essentials of life. Without enough water, the cells cannot function properly. Water is essential for detoxification, because our bodies eliminate most waste products with the help of water—in urine, in feces, which need enough hydration to move, and also in sweat. Most people today are dehydrated not only from not drinking enough water, but also because many foods and drinks, especially caffeinated ones, soda, and alcohol, have a dehydrating effect.

The other basic raw material missing in the modern diet is fiber. Fiber from plants doesn't get absorbed into the body as a nutrient; instead, it "sequesters" or pulls toxins out of the lower intestine (colon) after they have been processed in the liver and sent there for elimination. Without a quantity of fiber, the toxins can sit in the intestines, irritating them, and getting reabsorbed back into the body.

Wildfires

Though "inflammation" is the buzzword in diet books and health magazines, most people understand just part of what it means. It is thought of as a localized area that is swollen, painful, red, and warmer than the areas around it. But inflammation is a survival mechanism of great complexity. Inflammation occurs when a set of chemicals in the blood are activated by something foreign or broken. These chemicals attract defense cells that protect tissues against whatever is injuring them, from a thorn to a disease-causing microbe. The repair

Inflammation and Diet

"Fish oil" is one of the common names today for the essential omega-3 fats. But they don't only exist in fish; they exist in almost every living organism. Cows have plenty of these fats in their bodies when they live naturally, roaming free and eating grass. But when cows are confined to small spaces and fed corn, they become inflamed, generating excess amounts of omega-6 fats. Both omega fats and others are needed in the right proportion to sustain the balance of life.

This right proportion exists in nature; grass-fed cows have balanced ratios of them in their bodies, because they eat as nature intended. This balanced ratio no longer exists in the foods we eat—and therefore, in us. Unnaturally raised animals are inflamed

system is also activated by calling in different cells to fix the damage. Normally, inflammation is self-regulated, which means that as soon as it is triggered, it will start reactions that will stop further inflammation. However, if the body is constantly exposed to irritants, the inflammation response is switched on all the time—not just at small specific sites, but systemically all over the body and throughout the blood. This is what happens when exposure to toxins is high: modern humans are themselves. Even human consumption of plant food has contributed to this problem. Consider that our fertilizers are mostly made of three components, nitrogen, phosphorus, and potassium. Missing are all the others—selenium, zinc, magnesium, and manganese, to name a few of the fifty-two minerals that plants need to grow healthy. Plants are malnourished too. Their immune systems grow weak. When insects attack, plants respond with a defense mechanism of their own, getting inflamed. We created an inflamed society by eating inflamed plants, inflamed animals, and inflamed fish. We eat the inflammation when we consume the food we produce and, so, become it ourselves.

chronically inflamed. Inflammation (from the Latin word *inflatio,* "to set on fire") becomes to the body's environment what wildfires are to the planet's.

The body is built to work in harmony with nature, to make sure inflammation stays in check. It naturally sucks up certain nutrients from food that can switch inflammation on and off. An example of a nutrient that supports inflammation is omega-6 fatty acids; an example of one that switches it off, omega-3 fatty acids. These nutrients are designed by nature to exist in a balanced ratio everywhere, in our food and inside ourselves. Inflammation is not supposed to be left "on" for long, just neutral and always ready, if needed. Other essential anti-inflammatories such as polyphenols, curcumin, and MSM (methylsulfonylmethane) should be available in our diet.

A diet loaded with the anti-inflammatory nutrients could do the trick, even with the modern volume of toxins triggering the inflammation response. But without it, inflammation is "on" constantly. Soon, it is propagated throughout the body like the shockwaves of a grenade. It can become chronic and actually start degrading tissues, instead of fixing injuries. This lays the foundation for diseases like cancer, diabetes, and most notably cardiovascular disease. Clean is designed to boost your anti-inflammatory nutrients while reducing the triggers for inflammation to a large degree.

Melting Icebergs

When the organs of detoxification and elimination are overburdened and undersupported, they cannot do their job for the rest of the body. Depending on which cells or organs are affected the most, different diseases will manifest: arthritis, cancer, heart disease, and so forth. Some diseases occur when a body with reduced detoxification ability starts recruiting other systems to perform secondary "emergency" duties to help, sometimes in the extreme. This is all part of its design to survive. Take osteoporosis, for example. When acidity is chronic due to a bad diet, the bones can get recruited. Acidity control is more urgent for the body than bone formation, because high acidity is more lethal than osteoporosis. So the bones compensate by releasing some of their naturally alkaline bone salts, like calcium and phosphorus, to buffer acidity in the blood.

A specialist might then prescribe an expensive drug to stimulate the osteoblasts (the cells that "manufacture" bone) or large doses of calcium to encourage bone strengthening. But none of this makes sense without reducing blood acidity at the same time. Without the right alkalinity in the blood, that calcium will not be assimilated into bone and may actually end up in the coronary arteries or joints. (Furthermore, calcium is not deposited in the bones without adequate levels of vitamin D, a test for which is rarely ordered by primary-care physicians.) This is why drinking milk is now understood by some to be the worse possible way to combat osteoporosis. Milk generates acidity, which in the long run causes bone loss—not bone formation, as the milk industry wants you to believe. But we should take it back one step, before the treatment, and start with the question, "Why is the patient acidic?"

QUANTUM TOXINS

Toxicity is not limited to the realm of food and chemicals. There is another kind of toxicity that is just as pervasive and influential on modern health—even though it's harder to measure or isolate. Toxic thoughts, toxic relationships, the undercurrent of anxiety that is almost an automatic by-product of making it in the modern American world—all these things are pollutants in that they disturb the peace and normal body functioning we were born to have. Although it doesn't come up on the EPA's list of worst environmental dangers and is still not fully recognized by many busy doctors in hospitals (as the lack of adequate therapies in them reveals), the stress of modern life is as much a toxin as the chemicals in our food, water, and air.

Today there is a constant assault on our attention that keeps the mind switched on at all times. There is more information circulating than at any other time in human history. (Even the TV news is no longer just an anchorperson sitting at a desk. Now it has three lines of ticker-tape information streaming across the bottom. Our attention is literally being divided.) Add to that the situation where we are all available for communication at all times (and in all time zones). Cell phones, Bluetooth headsets, e-mails, text messages, faxes—it has become almost taboo to ever be disconnected. On top of this we are so busy all the time, striving for great careers, great relationships, great children, great homes—the pressure to achieve has never been higher and has us living in a constant state of planning, working, trying. All this energy going on in the brain keeps it from being available where it is needed in the body. In fact we are a society of people barely aware of our bodies—which may be suffering and breaking down under our noses as we keep thinking and worrying.

It was incessant, negative, fearful thinking that started me on my journey of self-healing. I could somehow cope with my allergies, my weight gain, and my irritable bowels, but it was my toxic thoughts that stopped me in my tracks and made me look for a deeper understanding. The toxic food I was eating, the toxic schedules I was working by, and the toxic hospital environment, full of fear and frustration, within one of the most toxic cities in the world had taken a toll on my body. But it wasn't until my incessant worrying and the chest pain it generated got me wondering if I was having a heart attack that I began searching for a different solution. My initial experience with meditation gave me hope and a clear goal, to silence my mind. In my case, at that time, everything else took second place—propelling me onto that plane to India.

I am still working on that goal for myself. But whatever ability I have gained to quiet my own mind allows me to recognize a similar level of distraction and the constant loop of thinking and worry in my patients. It is rampant in modern life; unproductive thinking rules us and controls our lives. We get stuck not just in habits of eating that hurt us and drain the energy necessary for our body's needs, but stuck in incessant thought. It also drains energy and leaves us fatigued, worn down, and with a physical body deprived of the resources it needs to heal itself. I call the negative effects of stress "quantum toxins" because they exist outside of the scope of doctors' measuring tools. Stress finds many ways to manifest in body, behavior, and outlook, influencing eating patterns, addictions, and belief in our own potential to be (or never be) well. Quantum toxicity is without doubt one of the greatest obstacles to vibrant well-being. How did it become this way?

Quantum toxicity is not new. In fact, thousands of years before humans invented preservatives, antibiotics, hormones, fertilizers, or any chemicals whatsoever, detoxification was the main topic for some very influential people on our planet. Buddhism, one of the oldest spiritual paths, was described as a path of detoxification by the Buddha himself. Professor Robert Thurman, who teaches Tibetan Buddhism at Columbia University, is a dear friend and one of my teachers. He once explained it to me in this way:

> In the Buddhist Wheel of Life, the center has a circle in which there are three animals, a pig, a cock, and a snake, holding each other by the tail. The pig stands for the delusion or ignorance that says, "I am the real thing, the center of the universe, and the most important being in it, and the rest and all others are separate from me!" This deep conviction of the egoistic being places that being in the unwinnable situation of confrontation with the universe, which any single being has got to lose, sooner or later. Based on this perspective, the being wants to consume lots of the universe, to turn it into him- or herself, and this is called greed, represented by the cock. If possible, the being would devour the whole thing and then would no longer need to fear it. But the universe is infinite, so that never

succeeds. Also, based on the same perspective, the being fears others want to devour him or her and so becomes paranoid and seeks to repel them all, and this is called anger and hatred, symbolized by the snake.

These are the three poisons or toxins (Sanskrit trivisha) that make the unenlightened world go around, the samsara of endless suffering. In Indo-Tibetan medicine they correspond to phlegm, wind, and bile in the physical realm (the kapha, vata, and pitta body types), or more generally, cohesion, movement, and heat. Health for an unenlightened person is the balance of these poisons and energies—that is the best that can be achieved. But real health, durable and joyous, comes from detoxification, removal of the poisons by wisdom, insight into the true nature of reality, the experience of the self being one with the universe, filled with energy and bliss, not needing to be greedy, not fearing or hating anyone, but being joyfully compassionate to all, seen as ultimately the same as oneself and beautiful in their relative difference—just as one sees one's beloved child or lover or good friend. This is the true health of enlightenment.

Enlightenment as true health may seem unattainable for so many of us, but getting rid of the poisons that Buddha spoke of could be, from this point of view, more urgent than anything we can do at the level of food, drink, and natural cleaning products. Only when freed of delusion, greed, and anger can we return to an enlightened state in which we live with the knowledge that we already have everything we need. Only this will truly stop the rampant consumption and human-made madness of modern life.

As part of Clean, you will be invited to start a short daily meditation practice, a chance to unload some of this mental burden and explore the very beginning of what "real health, durable and joyous" may mean to you.

CHAPTER SIX

The Common Root of Dysfunction: Digging for Answers

W hen the leaves of a plant start looking sick, wise gardeners will dig out the root to take a look. Even though it is buried in the soil, hidden from view, gardeners know they must go to the root to find where most plant diseases begin. It does not surprise them that it was far away from the root, on the leaves, that the first symptoms appeared. They know that for the leaves to be healthy, they must receive nutrients from the roots, where they are absorbed from the soil. I learned this as a kid, watching the gardeners in my own backyard.

As I looked for answers and solutions to my own health issues, my journey also changed me from Western-trained specialist to open-minded doctor. As I started studying other traditions of healing, one concept kept cropping up in many of them: health and disease start in the intestines. This concept, which initially I did not understand, held the key that unlocked the answer I was looking for. Hidden, just like roots, our intestines absorb nutrients from food, our soil. Intestinal health plays a huge role in whether we get well-nourished. Toxicity, depression, irritable bowel syndrome, nutrient depletion, mucus, acidity, serotonin production— all these loose pieces of the puzzle became connected in a multilevel matrix that answered my questions about how and why.

Most people underestimate the importance of intestinal health. Other organs, such as the heart (the "king of the organs"), tend to get center stage. Yet as I learned, information on this system proved to be the missing link between my irritable bowel syndrome and my depression.

The human gut is similar to the root of a plant: both are hidden, both absorb water and nutrients, and when sick, both can show symptoms on organs far away, like the leaves and branches or the skin and hair. But hidden in this root is one of the most important systems for human life: a high-precision machine with abilities and functions that not only allow us to obtain the building blocks and chemicals that will make our bodies, but also detect who to trust in life. A machine so delicate, it needs a very specific set of conditions for balanced function. Nature is the designer of the machine and also provided the perfect conditions. When we departed from the ways of nature, the conditions for optimal gut function deteriorated. When the intestines are in distress, nutrient deficiencies are likely. But also your intuition may suffer. Your "gut feelings" may get confused. Your seasonal allergies may come back with a vengeance. You may gain weight despite "not eating," get depressed, or get constipated. You may start to react to foods that you never reacted to before. Every single organ or function in the body has a direct link to the intestines.

Toxicity often affects the gut before any other organ. The gut, as I refer to it here, is not a single organ. It is a system that performs important, diverse, and almost magical functions. A short description of the four major constituents of the gut system will help you understand how it can be the root of the problem for totally different diseases.

THE INTESTINAL FLORA

The silent heroes of health, the beneficial bacteria that live in our intestines are so important that some healing traditions call them the "invisible organ." They may live far out of sight, but they are essential to the maintenance of intestinal integrity. A healthy intestine contains about two pounds of helpful bacteria. Like our inner rain forest, the intestines host a thriving mass of tiny microorganisms. These guests occupy prime real estate, cozy within the folds of the intestinal mucosa, our first skin. The rent is high, and they pay it in hard labor. They help with digestion, enabling essential nutrients to be absorbed that otherwise would have not been able to cross the intestinal wall into the circulatory system. The depletion of healthy intestinal flora guarantees nutrient depletion and its consequence, system malfunction. They also protect us from infections. They take up all the real estate on the intestinal walls so that other organisms, such as pathogenic flora (disease-causing bacteria), viruses, and parasites literally cannot get a foothold. From their prime location on the intestinal wall, the beneficial flora functions as the first filter for toxins, neutralizing about a quarter of them before they get inside the bloodstream. And their presence speeds up transit time of toxic waste in the colon (feces) so it doesn't sit there too long, which would let toxins get reabsorbed into the bloodstream.

There are always a few bad or pathogenic bacteria in this mix—it's inevitable. But modern living has altered this balance in almost everyone. Toxic chemicals, medications, and especially antibiotics—medicine designed specifically to kill "biota," or tiny life-forms—wipe out the good flora over time. Alcohol and stress contribute. The pathogenic or disease-causing microbes, resistant to the chemical mix that killed the good ones, find a way to survive and take over, a situation called dysbiosis. Yeasts are one of the organisms that overgrow the first chance they get. They thrive on the sweet foods and dairy products we eat and expel their waste, a toxic emission that makes *us* bloated, gassy, and irritated. Dysbiosis affects everyone to some extent—even those who eat whole foods and take probiotics, because we are all exposed to toxicity.

Many studies show the importance of good intestinal flora for all aspects of health. Mothers who take probiotics give birth to children who don't get sick and years later even do better in school. Athletes with healthy intestinal flora recover faster from injury. Meanwhile, taking antibiotics as a kid correlates significantly with having all kinds of diseases later on. In the toxicity story, this is such an important player that to embark on detox without restoring the good bacteria and removing the bad is almost pointless. Rebuilding, reinoculating, and restoring the intestinal flora will be an integral part of your Clean program.

Ironically, when I prescribe probiotics, other cardiologists look at me, puzzled. None of the hospitals I have worked in during my career had a useful stock of them, nor did I ever see them prescribed in other departments, although hospitals are arguably where they're needed the most. Even gastroenterologists, those who specialize in digestive organs, are only now looking at probiotics as a way to help their patients. Barely a thought is given to the condition of the animal population of the "inner forest."

New medical-grade probiotic brands are being developed by the pharmaceutical industry, targeted toward those with bloating, constipation, and irritable bowel syndrome. Even though it is a step in the right direction, the probiotics are still made and marketed by those with the same mind-set used with traditional drugs—as a magic-bullet cure to a complex problem. Their marketing suggests that damaged intestinal flora can be fixed with a probiotic product alone—no dietary changes or detox program is advised or even mentioned as helpful. This "one-stop shopping" approach is appealing, because it suggests we don't have to sacrifice anything to regain health. But it's counterproductive. Only when you eliminate the foods that feed the pathogenic bacteria, use natural antimicrobial foods or supplements to scare them off, and pro-

Antibiotic Overload

Science has done a great job of studying toxic bacteria that cause disease. It has succeeded in developing powerful weapons to kill them—antibiotics—which have saved many lives. But it has ignored the fact that killing the bad bacteria also kills the good flora that we need to thrive. The indiscriminate use of antibiotics has obliterated intestinal flora and contributed to everything from malnutrition and depression to infections by decimating this first line of defense. Now, the mutation of a number of these bad bacteria into dangerous and disease-causing superbugs, like the "hospital superbug" MRSA (methicillin-resistant Staphylococcus aureus), which is killing patients in the very place they come to get healed, is a result of the overuse of antibiotics.

vide live bacteria of the right strains and in the right number can you truly rebuild the intestinal flora successfully. Taking a pharmaceutical probiotic while continuing to drink coffee and eat doughnuts is like throwing a Tic Tac at a charging elephant.

The intestinal flora also helps with the in-house training of the body's inner Department of Homeland

Security. Because our intestinal first skin is the border with the most foreign visitors, which are all trying to get *in*, the immune system has built many military bases on the intestinal wall itself, with periscopes looking into the intestinal tube, where the good bacteria are fighting their battles and completing their work. The good bacteria, by teasing them, keep the guards alert enough to recognize any real threats, but not so much that they generate a state of alert, which would start recruiting all the services of the immune army all throughout the body. Around the intestinal tube, there are so many immune-system operation camps that all together they make up to 80 percent of the total immune system in the body. Gut-associated lymphatic tissue, or GALT, is the name it goes by. My prediction is that we will find many more functions performed by the GALT once researchers become interested.

THE INTESTINAL WALL

To get inside the body, inside the circulatory system, the bloodstream, anything foreign has to pass a border, a barrier that separates the inside of the body from the outside. The first skin, whether facing out (skin) or facing in (intestinal wall), needs to be intact to serve its protective purpose, that of filtering what gets inside. Whatever makes it to the inside must be chosen and transported on purpose (absorption) by the intestinal-wall cells themselves, the "bricks" of the wall. In a healthy intestine, the wall is smooth, with no cracks between the bricks. They have what are called "tight junctions." Such "tightness" is seen clearly under the microscope, and it serves an important purpose, to let *nothing* unwanted in.

The following is a simple way to think about a complex subject. Our body is designed to protect its inside from anything that doesn't belong there, anything foreign. For this purpose, there is a full army with different battalions and a host of weapons. One of the most delicate aspects of its intricate operation is the accurate identification of "self" and "foreign." Everything alive is made of the three basic bricks, carbohydrates, proteins, and fats (and a few other things such as water, metals, minerals, and salts). These in turn are made of amino acids (protein), carbon and water (carbohydrates), and fatty acids (fats). The whole universe is like a Lego set. Just a few different types of individual pieces, when joined together in different numbers and different arrangements, make billions of things so different it's hard to imagine that the building blocks are the same.

When we eat a piece of chicken, the digestive system gets to work. The job is to disassemble that chunk of chicken into its individual components. These are small enough to pass through the intestinal wall into the blood. Once in the blood, these components will not be stopped. It is impossible for the immune system's secret police to know if an individual component comes from a chicken, a nut, or an energy bar. It will soon be used to build something, possibly muscle.

But when a clump of components that are still attached (incompletely digested) and big enough to be recognized as a piece of chicken makes it through the wall, the alarm is almost instant, and a "shock and awe" type of response is launched. One type of immune cell (lymphocyte) shoots a glue (antibodies) that tags the foreigner (antigen) and stuns it. Killer cells are recruited and on arrival attach themselves to the foreigner and release on it acid juices so corrosive that they dissolve everything on contact.

Toxicity is at the root of the chain of events that ends with a damaged intestinal wall, with holes, so that it is not impermeable anymore to chunks of food. This is called "leaky gut," and the common set of symptoms and problems that result, the "leaky gut syndrome." The first skin is constantly renewing itself, and any gaps, injury, or damage will be repaired by growing cells and connective tissue much faster than usual until it is fixed. The bricks used to build the intestinal wall are not so readily available to begin with (glutamine), but in an environment like the one that caused a leaky gut, chances are the wall will never be repaired. To create the right conditions for your intestines to be able to get the repair they need is why I designed the Clean program.

GUT-ASSOCIATED LYMPHATIC TISSUE (GALT)

One of the families of diseases most puzzling to the Western medical world is the autoimmune diseases. These are diseases in which the immune system attacks areas of the body itself, an act of self-destruction. How and why would a system that was designed solely to distinguish between "self" and "foreign" get so confused that it orders its army to open fire on itself?

When the beneficial intestinal flora is killed by a mix of antibiotics, preservatives, coffee, and alcohol, more aggressive, resistant, and damaging bacteria occupy its space. The GALT now mounts all types of responses (allergic, defense, inflammatory, repair), triggered by these toxic bacteria and the chemicals in food. But when the intestines leak identifiable undigested pieces, the immune system goes full force. Never in the evolution of the body did it experience such intense attack. It does not have a system in place to select its battles. Every undigested chunk will keep triggering a full army attack.

Imagine an army with soldiers who were trained for only one or two battles at a time. Suddenly millions of calls are arriving from different locations for different battles. Soldiers run in circles and end up shooting anything that resembles a chunk of food. If the chunk under attack is from the muscle of a chicken, it is possible that the soldiers will end up shooting the muscle of the body they are designed to defend, because chicken muscle and human muscle are similar. (This is an imaginary scenario—I don't actually know of chicken muscle causing an immune attack on human muscle because of a leaky gut.)

What is not imaginary is that autoimmune diseases are on the rise. One of the earliest and most familiar autoimmune diseases is rheumatic fever. Strep in the throat generates a massive army deployment. Strep molecules have a surface similar to the surface of the valves in the heart, especially the mitral valve, and also to the large joints. The army mistakes the joints and heart valves for the strep and the fire is targeted at them. The joints recover, but the heart valve is damaged, scarred for life. Open-heart surgery for valve repair or replacement is often needed decades later.

Simply from exposure to the standard American diet, our GALT tends to live in a high state of alert, constantly initiating immune responses. This subtly steals

Living in a State of Red Alert

The good flora on the intestinal lining lives in harmony with the GALT. It keeps the immune-system tissue stimulated just enough to keep it ready for action at all times, without making it jump into defense mode. This is why healthy intestinal flora is key to healthy immunity, including ordinary defense against all kinds of colds and bugs. When your intestinal flora is ravaged, one of the first things you will notice is an increase in common colds and longer battles with sore throats and the flu, something that many people consider a "normal" part of what is now known as "cold season" (primarily because medication marketing has called it that). But it's not normal. A person with a highly functioning immune system, supported by healthy intestinal flora, will rarely get these illnesses. On the other hand, those whose intestines are colonized by bad bacteria are in a state of constant warfare, because the GALT can sense the pathogens living just above it. These people are much more likely to have allergies and inflammation throughout the body.

energy from the body's economy, which then has less energy available for healing, detoxification, and other important functions. This draining of energy reserves can be felt in many subtle ways including, obviously, daily tiredness.

When intestinal integrity is lost, the GALT is exposed to visitors that it would have never met under natural conditions. Foods that never posed a problem before may turn, under the conditions of toxicity, into potential allergens. The allergic-response army goes into red alert and sends signals to other parts of the body.

When you allow the body to repair the intestinal wall, replant good bacteria, and soothe the immune-inflammatory armies with specific nutrients, you could return to the times where reading a restaurant menu didn't feel like walking on a landmine field. You never know what step will detonate the blast.

OUR SECOND BRAIN

"Go with your guts," our wise advisers tell us. Our instant "gut instinct" is usually right about situations and people. It's our mind that messes things up and causes us to end up doing the things that our guts so clearly told us not to. "I should have listened to my guts," we lament later. Perhaps this function is what helped early men and women survive.

Around the intestines and GALT there is a well-kept secret—millions of nerve cells, almost as many as in the brain. This means an ability to process information about what's going on and put a response into action separate from the brain and central nervous system. The intestines can control their functions independent of the brain if necessary. And when it comes to the most important decisions in life, especially life and death, it's the intelligence of the intestines that we want to depend on, not the insecure, indecisive thinking brain.

The intestines can also take emergency action on their own: everyone knows how fear can cause an explosive contraction of the peristaltic machinery, sometimes causing diarrhea. This reflex is likely designed to prioritize energy in emergency situations. If confronted with a lion, you don't want to be spending your body's energy digesting. You'd want to instantly gather energy to fight or flee. So the body just dumps whatever food was keeping it busy in the name of survival.

The nerve cells in the intestines communicate with each other in the same way that brain neurons do, through chemicals called neurotransmitters. There are many kinds of neurotransmitters. Some are involved in excitation responses, others inhibitory responses.

Special Guests: Parasites

Eric, a successful movie actor, came to see me with two problems that don't go down well in Hollywood. He had eczema, or irritated, scaly skin, on the side of his face that no creams or medications could help. He was also "puffed up" with a few extra pounds. During his cleanse, Eric dropped about twelve pounds and he began to feel much better. His eczema calmed down until the end of his cleanse, when it returned in full force. Mystified, I suggested we get a stool test done to look for clues. Experience has shown me that when an otherwise healthy person continues to have mysterious symptoms after the Clean program is completed—whether they are skin issues, ongoing nausea, tiredness, constant bloating, or a general weakened state—there is an important next step. I look for the bug.

Parasites are organisms that live in the intestines and actively degrade your well-being by stealing nutrients. They mainly get in through food and water, often in restaurants, where there are more avenues for contamination, and they are common in many people who eat out a lot. (They are not just picked up on foreign trips, as most people think.) The clue that parasites are in residence is high inflammation, because the immune system is aggravated by their presence and initiates a fight. Eric's blood test showed a high CRP, one of the inflammation markers, so I asked him to visit a parasite expert for a consultation. The expert used rectal swabs to confirm the presence of parasites.

There are natural remedies for parasites that can be made at home and used during and after the basic three-week Clean program. Some of these are effective, such as eating ground-up papaya seeds daily, but Eric decided he wanted to take an aggressive approach. In this case, antibiotics and antiparasitics are the most effective treatment. We talked about the fact that this medication would damage his healthy intestinal flora, and he would need to work hard to replenish it afterwards with probiotics and good diet. Eric found that over the ten days of this program his skin symptoms finally disappeared for good. With the elimination of the parasites, his inflammation level went down, and the irritated skin, which was his body's way of showing him something was wrong, went away. With the invaders removed, balance was restored in his intestinal ecosystem and he could bloom again. Parasites are not addressed directly by the Clean program, but it may become relevant to your own search for balance if specific problems persist.

One of the most well known is serotonin, thought to be the responsible for the feeling of happiness and well-being. The popular theory is that it gets made in the brain, because it determines our moods and emotions. Not surprisingly, I discovered that an estimated 80 to 90 percent of the total amount of serotonin in our bodies is manufactured by the nerve cells of our gut. The gut system performs four functions: getting information from the outside world, engulfing components to be used in building of our organs and tissues, sensing the signals in the realm of intuition, and border patrol.

When toxicity damages the gut system, the entire economy of the body changes. Attention is directed toward fighting the pathogens and bacteria and generating immune and inflammatory responses. Meanwhile, the bad bacteria and yeast are actually competing for many of the nutrients needed for the manufacture of neurotransmitters and other substances essential for the proper functioning of our bodies, including serotonin. It's a battle for resources. When raw materials are scarce, your serotonin levels go down. Other neurotransmitters, like the ones that cause stress responses (adrenalin, noradrenalin), can then take center stage. As you will read, serotonin doesn't just affect psychological moods. It affects the "mood" of your bowels, which is why disrupted serotonin production contributes to both irritable bowels and depression.

DIG THE WELL BEFORE YOU ARE THIRSTY

Chinese medicine sees the human being as part of the one unbroken wholeness called the Tao. It strives to protect the balance of our internal ecosystem through diet, herbs, and modalities such as acupuncture, so that order is maintained and sickness doesn't get a chance to set in. A famous text written in the second century BCE says, "To cure disease after it has appeared is like digging a well when one is already thirsty or forging weapons after the war has already begun." Our current modus operandi in the West involves digging a lot of wells when we are already thirsty. And it's not working to keep us truly "well."

Outside of medicine, there is a shift in the markets. The natural-foods industry has exploded. The spread of the organic lifestyle beyond food has resulted in innovative products for every room of a greener, cleaner home. You can get water filters for your home and air filters for your car. You can stock your cupboards with supplements, herbal remedies, and put green cleaning products under the sink.

These measures are important. Reducing exposure today is the first step to building health for tomorrow. But unfortunately these innovations alone aren't enough. Even those making good lifestyle choices still shower with city water, eat food prepared by restaurants, and go into buildings that have been cleaned and fumigated with toxic chemicals. They may do the best they can, but they are susceptible to toxins from many areas that are outside of their control.

Preventive measures and well-designed eco-products improve the present and future, but they can't undo the past. Because of the stubbornness of certain human-made toxins, which tend to linger inside the body for years, the damage on the inside is already done or is in progress.

In an era when heart disease, an almost entirely avoidable condition, is the number-one killer in our country; when a staggering portion of the American GNP is used to pay for drugs and treatments for the so-called diseases of civilization; when the percentage of men and women who use prescription drugs daily is sky-high and growing, especially among those in midlife and older; one kind of future is laid out before you, one of ever-worsening health and a diminishing sense of well-being. Why not choose a different future, by digging the well now, when you have the strength to dig deep—before you have been further weakened?

That well is Clean, a tool for cleaning up the polluted inner environment, slowing down the rate of aging, and releasing the toxic overload that blocks optimal body functioning—now and in the future. Detoxification programs are not the panacea for every ill, but they help create a better state of health and give you back the power over your own well-being.

ARE YOUR GENES YOUR "DESTINY"?

Our genes contain all the information we need for life. Like the software in your computer, your genetic blueprint has the step-by-step instructions to manufacture your proteins, hormones, and everything else that your body needs to build itself as well as to repair itself and adapt to the changing environment and circumstances. The general public's current understanding is that there is little you can do if you inherit "bad genes."

Some genes are fixed in their effect, like the genes that determine the color of your eyes, but many more can be turned on or off. "Expression" is the key word here. Genes can be expressed or not expressed. The mechanics are something like this. We know now that far more information is contained in our genes than whatever is being used at any given moment. Like the software in your computer, some of the programs are running all the time, while other programs are dormant and run only when needed, when we click on them and open them for a specific purpose. Some genes contain the exact opposite of the information possessed by the gene right next to it. Our cells have developed a way to keep some of these genes dormant, inactive, unexpressed, while putting others to use. When the circumstances require it, some of the genes that are active can be turned off and the inactive ones turned on, or "expressed." The functions that they govern may be needed only at certain times, so when they are not needed they are in standby mode.

Expression of Genes

What determines whether and when a gene is expressed? The condition of your inner environment, your inner climate, is thought to be a major influence on triggering or suppressing genes that can cause disease. Genes are located in the nuclei of cells. The cytoplasm of the cell surrounds the nucleus, from where genes direct the symphony of life. The microclimate in the cytoplasm affects the genes. And what influences the cytoplasm of the cell? The blood surrounding the cell.

What influences the composition of the blood? The food you eat, the emotions you're having, the thoughts you are thinking, and the toxins you are accumulating. All these different influences have the potential to turn genes on and off. Mental or emotional states, environmental influences such as heat, humidity, light, sound, and others, radiation, even the perception of a loving nurturing environment as opposed to a threatening one have been shown to influence which genes get activated, resulting in different molecular processes. Of all the influences, the impact of food on our inner chemical environment is the most intimate one. After all, we are introducing it into our blood. The science that studies how our food affects the way our genes express themselves is called nutrigenomics.

Using what we know about our genes, we can make diet and lifestyle choices that will maximize the expression of our full potential and minimize the expression of genes that make us vulnerable or sick. For example, researchers at Johns Hopkins University recently discovered that sulforaphane, a sulfur-containing compound found in the seeds of broccoli, toned down the expression of certain cancer genes. They extracted this compound from broccoli seeds and turned it into a supplement that shows great promise in preventing cancers.

What nutrigenomics shows is that food not only "becomes what you are" by providing the building blocks for your bodily architecture, but also very closely directs which products of your metabolism will be increased and which will be decreased or stopped altogether. It can affect genetic expression for the better or the worse. In addition to saying, "We are what we eat," it seems as though we have to add, "Our cells behave the way our foods direct them to behave." Food brings information about our surroundings to the doors of our Pentagon, the GALT. If our surroundings are inflamed, then maybe food informs the intestines to prepare for the aggressor.

Nutrigenomics gives hope to people with the "genes equals destiny" perception. We have known for a long time that if people live healthy lives, they can neutralize the effects of certain genes that they inherited from their ancestors. Greater genetic predisposition for disease does not have to mean a guarantee of actually suffering from the disease. Nutrigenomics gives us a more powerful way to change our own future.

Doctors can identify certain genetic tendencies through some simple information gathering; for example, if one of your parents had a heart attack before age fifty, you are far more likely to have one yourself. With educated lifestyle choices you can minimize the chances that this will occur. Gene activation and deactivation may take too long to save your life if you are having a heart attack already. In this case, more immediate results may be needed. Medications, procedures, and tests will keep you alive in the short term. Eventually, if you want a long-term solution, you will need to turn genes off. A sound detox program is a great way to initiate this process.

With the Clean program you optimize your genetic expression in a simple and effective way. By changing your metabolism and reducing your blood acidity, your inflammation levels, your stress levels, and the toxins you are exposed to, you are improving that crucial environment in the cells on which genetic expression depends.

Your Genes Can Tell Your Doctor How to Write Your Prescriptions

Individual gene variation explains why the current "one dose for all" approach to prescribing medications is useless half the time and dangerous the rest. There are very small components of the DNA strand, the nucleotides, that have a big job. A certain kind of nucleotide, when present in the gene, signals the production of a liver enzyme that accelerates the metabolism of specific prescription medications. The presence or absence of this single nucleotide variety explains why some people bleed to death while others develop clots on the same dose of a blood-clotting inhibitor.

When this nucleotide is absent, the same medication may take ten times as long to be eliminated. This increases the chances of overdosing. Depending on the medication in question, it can be life-threatening. Such small differences in people's genes are called SNPs (single nucleotide polymorphisms). Deciphering their message is allowing a personalized, individualized approach to treatments. Gene testing that reveals this information is available, but not yet covered by health-insurance policies. The high cost of DNA testing is bound to drop, a trend that will support this direction in medicine.

CHAPTER SEVEN

The Clean Program

Whenever I see a new patient, at our first meeting we spend an hour or more talking about the person's present state of health. Frequently patients tell me they have been diagnosed with a disease and have been given prescription medications, mostly to alleviate their symptoms. Before I agree with any diagnosis, I tell my patients that their symptoms are the way their bodies and minds are telling them that things are not really working. Whatever they are doing, eating, and thinking has created an imbalance and their body is screaming at them that something needs to change. We are designed by nature to survive and procreate, and we have evolved to do so incredibly successfully over millennia. So the symptoms they are feeling are part of evolution's most powerful and sophisticated driving force, survival. To kill the symptoms without changing the conditions that caused them is insulting to the body's intelligence.

Some symptoms do point to immediate life-and-death situations, in which case emergency measures are needed to preserve life. For acute situations, modern medicine has developed life-saving technologies that are nothing short of miraculous. As a cardiologist I know that chest pain moving into the left arm classically happens when a clot stops blood from flowing through the arteries that feed the heart muscle. In this emergency scenario, catheters can be guided inside the arteries, from the groin up into the heart, to confirm this diagnosis and to allow doctors to break the clot by blowing up balloons that will stretch the arteries open. Science fiction has nothing more impressive than a modern cardiac catheterization lab, where saving lives is the daily routine.

But most patients' complaints are not indications that something is really "broken" and endangering their lives. The great majority of physical symptoms point to problems that would take much longer to cause death. These are symptoms of the chronic diseases that, according to statistics, most Americans will present with, sooner or later and to varying degrees, in their lifetime. These are the diseases that cost so many so much suffering and money. For these chronic ailments and their related symptoms, modern medicine has little to offer. The wonder chemicals and surgeries that are so effective in emergencies are the cause of worse suffering or even death when used to silence symptoms long-term.

I believe that whatever health problem is affecting my patients, their incredibly intelligent body will attempt to survive. The mechanisms it puts to work in order to do that get confused with the disease. Symptoms are the alarm system that makes us aware and demands we try something different from whatever we're currently doing—since that was what got us into trouble to begin with. To expect different results from doing the same thing is the definition of madness.

Instead of blocking the symptoms with medication, I try to answer the question, "What is it that my patient is trying to survive?" Something doesn't add up. We have split the atom and broken the genetic code, yet our society is sicker that it has ever been. What are we missing?

THE NATURAL ABILITY TO HEAL

The human body has an amazing natural ability to defend, repair, heal, and even rejuvenate itself. It is the magic you would see if you were to look at a magnified, high-speed movie of a cut on your skin. You would see that the bleeding stops when corklike bundles of cells, blood platelets, stop the bleeding by clumping up and filling up the blood vessels where they are cut, but nowhere else. And then, as if guided by an invisible hand, the skin cells on each border of the cut would start dividing and bridging the gap, until the whole surface was covered by skin, and the cut completely vanished, leaving just a reminder—a scar.

I tell my patients that even though they can't see it, the healing process is the same under the skin, deep inside the body. When damage occurs inside a healthy body, a number of mechanisms are triggered that are perfectly designed to stop the insult and then repair the damage, provided the conditions they need to complete the work are available. If they are not, the healing process fails and symptoms persist or worsen.

Two basic problems are responsible for the loss of this ability, resulting in chronic disease:

1. Obstacles that block cell functioning and chemical reactions
2. Lack of the ingredients needed for this process to occur

Modern Medicine's Blind Spot

When I look at what is happening with a patient's health, I ask myself these questions:

> What was the original insult that caused irritation or injury?
> What obstacles are preventing the body from healing?
> What is lacking that is needed to repair things?

The answer to the first two questions is often the same: the toxic overload we are exposed to in our daily lives. The air we breathe, the water we drink and shower with, the buildings we live and work in, the cosmetics we use, and the foods we eat are loaded with chemicals that alone or in combination damage our bodies and every other living creature on this planet. The chemicals we prescribe actually worsen the toxic burden we intend to correct.

Toxicity irritates tissues, damages our own cells, and kills other cells that we host in harmony and need for our health. When our body attempts to defend itself and repair the damage, toxins are often the obstacles that prevent it. The toxins bind to useful chemicals and prevent them from doing their work.

They irritate cells persistently, forcing the inflammatory, allergic, and defense mechanisms to act longer and more intensely.

Minerals, vitamins, and other nutrients in our foods is the answer to the third question. All the chemicals needed for our body chemistry and architecture would be provided by nature if we respected its ways. Comfort and greed drove us to change nature's design for growing plants and animals, resulting in a severe depletion of the nutrients that our body needs to function. Mass agriculture in exhausted soils produces plants that are depleted. Then we irradiate them, wax them, and turn them into all kinds of products that are loaded with toxins such as preservatives and additives. Growing cattle, chicken, and fish on an industrial scale has resulted in massive toxicity as well.

For all these reasons food lacks essential nutrients and turns out to be the biggest source of toxic chemicals. When you add the thousands of other chemicals of modern life, as well as the toxic influences invisible to the naked eye (thoughts, emotions, radiation), you have the perfect recipe for chronic diseases.

Whether toxicity is the primary or secondary cause of illness, it seems to be an integral part of the disease equation, since nobody is able to escape it completely. Everything is connected in such an intricate way, often with so many points between first cause and ultimate effect, that it is impossible to map every reaction. The time has come when we are waking up to an alarming truth. We are killing ourselves with the same chemicals we invented to make life easier. This concept has never been more relevant than in our modern life, yet so under the radar of our collective awareness. Until now.

What Is Cleansing?

Cleansing is turning up the intensity and effectiveness of the detoxification system. Supporting the process with the right nutrients is safe cleansing. Going beyond this to also promote the repair of the gut system is the essence of Clean.

Cleansing and detoxification programs may be returning to popularity today, but they are certainly not new to humans. Every ancient system of health care had ways of regularly attending to the body's detoxification systems and making sure the lines of defense in the body were working properly—and this was centuries before industrial chemicals filled the air. Humans have always instinctually known that a regular period of resting and recharging the body will let it shed the accumulated toxins and waste materials that tend to build up in all of us simply from living. It is also a way to boost healing when systems are taxed and are beginning to show signs of stress.

Every creature in nature does this periodically, alternating cycles of growth and activity with cycles of rest, such as hibernation. This keeps things in balance. Animals stop consuming food when they get sick. They rest the digestive system, so that energy can be diverted toward defense and healing.

As I learned during my own time in India, the Sanskrit word "Ayurveda" can be translated as the science of longevity. Its core philosophy is that health is a state in which the body is clear of toxins, the mind is settled, emotions are happy, wastes are constantly eliminated, and organs are working efficiently. To achieve this goal, Ayurvedic doctors give their patients balancing diets and herbs as part of a treatment plan. But they also prescribe regular periods of deeper detoxification known as *panchakarma,* during which the patients follow a cleansing program for several weeks and have hands-on treatments to pull toxins out of tissues and quiet the busy mind. This was developed millennia before smokestacks and diesel trucks arrived on the scene. Ayurveda understands that a part of ordinary human experience is the tendency to build up waste and accumulate stress, and if we don't spend some time alleviating this at a deeper level, our systems and organs get fatigued, making us sick.

Chinese health care is similarly wise. Frequently Chinese doctors put their patients on a program of teas, tonics, and treatments to help them throw off the toxins and mental fatigue they accumulate just by eating, breathing, and meeting everyday demands. Native Americans and members of other indigenous cultures around the world have used fasting and sweat lodges to purify body, mind, and spirit. Done periodically, the sweat-lodge experience returns participants to a path of clarity on every level, or is used strategically to heal disease.

All these traditions know that the simple experience of being human brings with it the need to periodically focus on cleansing and detoxifying. When we consider the weight of our modern toxic load and its taxing effects on our inner environments, a period of detoxifying practically becomes obligatory.

It's important to distinguish between a detox program (a cleanse) and the more generalized practice of slowly "cleaning up our act" by making gradual diet or lifestyle changes over several months. A cleanse is a distinct program, done for a concentrated period of time, that puts the body in a more intense detox mode. It has a start and an end date and a specific purpose.

These kinds of detoxification programs have also long been valued as a chance for the mind to come back to a peaceful center. In ancient times, cleansing through fasting was used as a tool to gain spiritual clarity. Cleaning out the *amma* wasn't just about diet; it was a process of cleansing the spirit of the toxic feelings and thoughts that cause suffering in the heart and soul. Jesus fasted for forty days and forty nights; Muhammad, Gandhi, and Buddha all fasted. Fasting for ultimate clarity about the nature of life is a part of many spiritual traditions and has been ingrained in humans for thousands of years.

For most people living busy lives today, the primary motivation to cleanse and detoxify is to remove the heaviness, fog, or lack of energy that is a consequence of contemporary lifestyles and stress. But dig a little deeper and there's often an underlying eagerness to simplify and strip away excess for a period of time, make some space, and get a new start by taking leave of some old, stuck patterns. There is an inevitable awakening in the mind and emotions, even if the stated goal of the cleanse is more physical, such as to enhance beauty, encourage weight loss, or look younger.

Health care in the twenty-first century is in the process of being radically reinvented. Ancient methods of protecting and preserving body and mind are being integrated with new discoveries in biochemistry and quantum physics. A new era of detox programs is being born. Clean sets the standard, for its design intentionally addresses both ingredients of good cleansing practices: the elimination of toxins and the repair of the gut.

How Clean Works

Everywhere I look today, there is growing curiosity about cleansing. As information is exchanged between individuals and as articles and tips are posted online about the many methods for detoxifying, there's more confusion than ever. It can be overwhelming. Descriptions of extreme programs can deter people from starting. Also people often get disillusioned a few days in, when the program they've selected turns out to be incompatible with their needs or simply uncomfortable. Sometimes the program they've picked can even be dangerous.

When we understand that a cleanse is a way of harnessing the body's natural intelligence, we learn that we can drive it in specific ways. Picking one type of cleanse-detox program over another is really about adjusting the intensity and speed of detoxification to best suit our bodies and lifestyles while we do it. Clean is a comprehensive program designed for the daily requirements of the busy lives we lead. There are benefits that happen quickly and I urge you to do the best you can. If for any reason one week of the program is the limit you can accomplish on the first try, you will still see and feel a difference. Perhaps next time one week can turn into two weeks or even the complete program.

Assessing the different methods of cleansing is a complex challenge. It becomes easier when you consider three pivotal factors:

- How intensely does the detox program switch the body into detox mode?
- How much nutritional support does it offer while the detox process is taking place?
- Does the program create the conditions for repair of the gut?

Though you don't need an advanced degree in medicine to proceed, it's helpful to understand what happens during the Clean program. For this, it's important to look at the mechanics of detoxification and how we harness this natural mechanism and boost it during a detox program.

The detoxification function is a joint venture of many organs and systems that work in harmony to neutralize and eliminate toxins, both "inner," the by-products of normal metabolism, and "outer," toxins we eat, breathe, or absorb through our skin and intestines. The function involves the liver, the intestines, the kidneys, the lungs, the skin, and the blood and lymphatic circulatory systems. It's an extraordinary system of great complexity and brilliant design.

DETOXIFICATION: AN ALL-DAY ACTIVITY

Though you probably never give it much thought, at every moment of every day your cells are breathing, working, and generating waste. It is part of the basic formula of life: your body is constantly performing an unimaginable number of functions every single instant of your living existence.

Each of the trillions of cells that make up your body is like a miniature factory that manufactures a product, from hormones to cartilage, hair, enzymes, protein, serotonin, and many more. Sugar from food and oxygen from air are what each cell factory uses for power. Sugar is burned to release energy. It also generates waste that must get thrown out. The waste is released into the circulatory system and then captured downstream by

The Web of Waste

Inner waste is constantly being eliminated to ensure your survival. You probably know that:

If you don't get rid of carbon dioxide, you asphyxiate.

If you don't get rid of uric acid, you can develop gout and heart disease.

If you don't get rid of homocysteine, from the breakdown of certain amino acids, you can develop Alzheimer's and heart disease.

If toxins in general are not handled in a timely manner, your inflammatory system goes into overdrive.

If you don't get rid of food debris, you can develop bowel disease—or at the very least, constipation.

On a subtler but still powerful level, if you don't get rid of anger or anxiety, it can manifest as heart disease, cancer, and many other kinds of bodily injury.

Detoxification in a healthy human is an intricate web of activities, guided by natural intelligence.

other cells whose function is to neutralize it. This process of neutralization makes these waste molecules nontoxic; now they can be safely filtered out of the body by the skin (as sweat), the lungs (as carbon dioxide), the kidneys (as urine), the liver (which mixes them with bile and releases them into the intestines), and the intestines directly (as fecal matter). Getting rid of waste is as critical to life as producing energy. Without it, waste products would accumulate and become so toxic that life would be terminated. Detoxification, therefore, is an ongoing activity that the body is brilliantly designed to accomplish.

THE BODY'S ECONOMY OF ENERGY

To understand detoxification, you have to become familiar with the body's energy economy. Energy is as precious a resource for your body as it is for the planet. The sum total of the energy expense of every cell is called *metabolism*. Each cell consumes fuel to make energy and then uses up that energy fulfilling its function. Thus, metabolism is *the energy cost of maintaining life.*

Some cells have functions that are more "expensive" than others—they cost more energy to run. Like a city with a financial budget to distribute on many city services, the body has an energy budget to spend. Energy reserves are limited, so the body must prioritize second to second how the energy capital gets distributed. If it spends too much energy in one area, it simultaneously has to cut back somewhere else to compensate. The body can't take out energy loans; when the energy reserves start running low, it has to stop activity. It might make you tired and sleepy, because when you rest and stop moving your muscles, you stop one of the costliest activities as far as energy goes.

Reallocating the Energy Cash Flow

Sometimes there are so many energy demands at once that split-second adjustments have to be made in what is basically an intricate balancing of the budget. The body's intelligence will shut down certain functions temporarily, slow down others, and allow the most crucial ones to continue spending their full energy "cash flow," since their function is deemed to be most vital. Neurons in the brain get top priority. As systems get shut down one by one, from least important to most, the brain is always the last. Without the brain, survival is over.

The body's detoxification processes lie somewhere in the middle of this list of priorities. It's very common for the body to put detox on hold, then catch up with cleaning later. For example, during hard exercise detox is put on hold. When muscles contract, they burn sugar in combustion with oxygen, and the waste product is carbon dioxide. The carbon dioxide dissolves in the blood as carbonic acid, circulates in the bloodstream, and when it enters the lungs, it is turned into a gas and exhaled. If the carbonic acid were not eliminated as carbon dioxide gas, it would accumulate in the blood, becoming so toxic that it would kill you faster than you can imagine.

But when you push into the harder exercise realm of anaerobic exercise—meaning you're burning sugar faster than oxygen can be taken in—you make a different waste product, lactic acid. Anaerobic exercise has an abnormally high energy expense, because the muscle is working so hard, and the body has to shift its energy distribution quickly to fund it. So it puts detoxification on hold, which is why lactic acid accumulates in the muscles. Knowing that the exercise won't go on for too long, the body lets it sit for a while and saves the expense of detoxifying it. (The side benefit is that, should that muscle go crazy for some reason and want to continue working at that level without stopping, the same lactic acid will irritate it so much that pain will eventually make the muscle stop. Muscle pain, in this case, is another survival mechanism.) Once the exercise stops,

The Real Energy Cost of Food

Food and the processes connected with it consume a big portion of our daily energy reserves. Digestion, absorption, the transportation of nutrients through the blood, and assimilation into the cells are highly expensive processes for the body. Not to mention growing, picking, and preparing the food—or working at a job to make money to buy it. In fact, some of the most energy-intensive functions of the body involve turning food into fuel and into the building blocks of the body's architecture. Sometimes we spend more energy processing food than we actually get from the food itself.

The whole process of digestion from start to finish has one of the highest energy costs in the body. Producing saliva costs energy. The production of enzymes consumes large amounts of energy. (During the Clean program you will increase the intake of enzymes by eating plenty of raw foods, thus conserving that energy and supporting digestion.) Muscles need energy to contract and push food to the stomach, which must then secrete digestive juices and push the mix through to the intestines. The pancreas and gallbladder meanwhile produce their signature substances—insulin and glucagon in the former case and bile in the latter.

Once the food has been broken down into small enough pieces, the molecules must be absorbed through the intestinal wall into the bloodstream. Now there's the work of transporting these building blocks to different sites in the body, where they can be assimilated by the cells and used to build your architecture, fund chemical reactions, and so on. This explains why the simple act of eating carries such a high energy cost.

Since modern habit is to eat frequently throughout the day, the constant energy requirement never stops. Often there is no energy left for anything else. Think of Thanksgiving dinners: the only activity possible after consuming all that food is to take a nap. Though everyone has a different theory explaining this dramatic drop in energy—from the tryptophan in turkey meat causing drowsiness to the alkaline blood currents that are generated as a result of producing excess acids in the stomach—the fact is that any big feast will put you to sleep, because digesting food takes a lot of energy. Every species of animal has this experience. Lions sleep for a few days after a big kill.

detoxification is immediately resumed, and the lactic acid is processed and transformed for elimination.

This pausing of detoxification to deal with other needs happens quite naturally in healthy bodies. Now add in the impact of the toxic overload of modern life, with its exotoxins, and it becomes clear why we all have a detox debt to varying degrees.

The Inner Economic Crisis

The energy expense of eliminating the toxins of daily life plus the added expense imposed by modern toxins causes a recalibration of the energy economy. If nothing else were going on, then cutting back on a little muscle movement and a couple of other not so vital expenses would probably compensate. But the demands are too big. We are drawing on our energy reserves to fund crazy work schedules, mental and emotional stress, and many more "extra" expenses that modern life imposes. The largest one of all is the digestion of food. Contrary to the assumption that food is where we *get* our energy from, modern life has turned the processing of foods by the body into a business that exacts the biggest energy drain. We are constantly eating and munching. Anything that we throw in *must* be processed when it arrives in the stomach—we can't put that off. But most of what we throw in today has minimal nutritional value, so all the energy we invest in its chewing, swallowing, digesting, and absorbing gives minimal return on investment. We are making less than we spend.

TRIGGERING THE SIGNAL: HOW WE ENTER DETOX MODE

Confronted with this huge load of demands, the body has to prioritize, redistribute, and reorganize. As long as digestion is using up so much of the energy budget, detoxification is partly on hold. All the extra modern toxins we're exposed to, having made their way into circulation and into the different tissues, will be retained where they are, just as lactic acid is retained in the muscles while the intense muscle work is going on. Since these extra toxins are irritants, the cells coat them with mucus to tone the irritation down while they anxiously wait for the signal from the body's central bank that energy is available for detoxification and it is okay to release these toxins back into the circulatory system.

In the case of lactic acid that has accumulated during intense anaerobic activity, the signal to start detox is sent when the muscle stops working. In the case of toxins that accumulate in the tissues, the detox signal is sent when digestion, absorption, and assimilation are completed. It is the green light for the body to enter detox mode.

A detoxification program is designed to trigger this signal more intensely than normal, principally by reducing the workload of the digestive tract. If digestion is stopped long enough and frequently enough, the signal to detox gets switched on more often and turned to "high." This initiates the release of accumulated toxins and the mucus that coats them. But it's only the beginning. Once the toxins are set free from the tissues they've lodged in, they are free to circulate in the blood. The "buffering" mucus coat falls off and circulates too. Both the toxins and the mucus must be rapidly neutralized and expelled, or they will cause damage to the body at large. Though toxins are harmful sitting in your tissues, coated with mucus, they can cause even more harm if released en masse and not treated. It's like liberating hundreds of prisoners into the city streets with no program of rehabilitation for them.

Detox Equalization

Cleansing and detox programs accelerate and enhance the removal of toxins. But the acceleration of the first action (toxin release) does not mean that the second action (neutralization) speeds up automatically to match it. The two processes occur through different mechanisms. That's why a successful and safe detox program requires that the two processes take place in a balanced way. Knowledge and experience are needed to equalize them, to avoid discomfort and even damage. This balancing of release and neutralization is what distinguishes the different styles of detox programs from each other as well as the speed at which intestinal-system damage is repaired.

DETOX PROGRAMS: THE BASIC MECHANICS

You finish the work of processing your food about eight hours after your last meal. Only then can the body turn its attention to "cleaning up" not only the day's mess, but also all the accumulated garbage that you have not had the energy or detox time to get to for weeks, months, or years (if not decades). Once digestion is done, the signal to release accumulated toxins from tissues into circulation (bloodstream and lymphatic system) can get triggered. Not every meal is created equal: quantity and quality of food may cause the signal to go on sooner, six hours after eating, or later, up to ten hours after the meal. As a general rule, the more you eat, the longer it takes to process your meal and for the signal to start intense detoxification.

Solid foods must first be liquefied for digestion; this takes energy and time. Liquid meals are practically ready for absorption, bypassing the need and energy expense of being broken down.

Cooked foods delay the detox signal further, because heating any food above 118° Fahrenheit destroys the enzymes contained in it. Enzymes are of paramount importance for digestion. Manufacturing them take so much energy that nature provides them already made. Raw vegetables, fruits, nuts, and seeds contain the enzymes necessary for their own digestion. When those foods get cooked, we lose that important resource. We have to manufacture all our own enzymes from scratch, which adds to the energy cost of eating and delays the funding for detoxification.

There are other factors influencing when, if, and how efficiently we enter detox mode. If we ingest a food that triggers an allergic response, a host of processes are put in motion that consume even more energy and time. When the GALT, the immune cells that live close to the intestinal wall, get irritated, they start manufacturing substances—histamines and immunoglobulins—to mediate allergy, which in turn activate a series of responses, including the activation of the inflammatory system. Thus, foods that cause allergies end up activating three bodywide systems: the digestive, immune, and allergic systems, all high energy consumers. When they're switched on, a snowball effect starts: one reaction triggers the next in a chain of reactions that recruit other cells and cause specific effects such as sneezing, itching, vomiting, vasodilatation, and more. By using up so much of the energy budget, they cause detoxification to get delayed even longer. And simultaneously, they cause disruption all over the body—draining resources further. The chaos and confusion caused by irritating foods can drain the body, the patient, and the doctors, who typically don't connect the problem to irritating foods or the eroded state of the intestines to the presenting symptoms. Pulling this picture into focus makes very clear how every one of us, over time, can end up with a backlog of toxins in our tissues.

The news is not all bad, though. Some foods delay the signal to start dumping toxins, but other foods accelerate it by supporting and enhancing the many steps in digestion and absorption. Magnesium-rich foods promote intestinal motility and accelerate intestinal transit. Olive oil facilitates transit by lubricating the walls as well as triggering the release of bile from the gallbladder. Bile is crucial for effective digestion. Enzyme-rich foods speed up the process by supplying the body with many of the enzymes needed. Nature actually provides much of what we need to get toxins out of our bodies, if we just follow its rules.

This understanding is the basis of an "Elimination Diet." Avoiding the foods that are difficult to digest and that are known to cause food allergies and sensitivities will allow the body to enter detox mode reliably and consistently. When you combine meals that follow the Elimination Diet guidelines with liquid meals, as you will do during the Clean program, you reduce the workload of digestion even further. Naturally, this helps the detox mode to start sooner, last longer, and consequently clean deeper.

DISARMING THE TOXINS: THE LIVER'S IMPORTANT WORK

The toxins and mucus that are released into circulation once detox mode has been switched on must get neutralized and eliminated. Why? Because these toxins contain free radicals, electrically charged molecules that corrode tissues and damage cells on contact. In addition, different toxins interfere with different functions such as cell division and reproduction, hormone assembling and release, and receptor sensitivity. And as described earlier, they even affect gene expression, altering the way our genes govern the inner workings of the body and literally changing the course of our life expression at the origin of command. Furthermore, since toxins, particularly the human-made ones, are by and large fat lovers (lipophillic), if they circulate long enough without being neutralized, they will find fatty tissue to lodge within. The brain, with its high percentage of fat, is a prime target. Neurological disturbances are, not surprisingly, a consequence of accumulated toxicity.

Because fat is hard to offload (as everyone knows), the newly freed toxins must get transformed from fat-soluble molecules into water-soluble molecules, which can be more easily excreted. The central player in this part of the story is the liver. Its cells contain a group of enzymes called the cytochrome P450 system, which are designed to cause the chemical reactions for this crucial process of neutralization. The reactions are performed in two steps, phase 1 and phase 2 liver detoxification. During phase 1, the structure of the toxin being neutralized is actually altered and it is turned into an "intermediate metabolite." In some cases, this intermediate product is more toxic than the toxin it came from. The rush is now on to push it through to the second phase of liver detoxification, which will neutralize the toxic property and transform it into a water-soluble product that can then be thrown back into blood circulation and passed through to the blood vessels inside the kidneys. The kidney cells will recognize it, capture it out of the blood, and finally release it into the urethra as urine. You pee it out and with this act of elimination, the detoxification journey is completed.

This essential liver work has some important requirements. It requires energy, a steady supply of antioxidants (to neutralize the free radicals), and an array of other minerals, vitamins, and nutrients (to feed the chemical reactions of phases 1 and 2). If all these things are available, detoxification occurs safely. The transition between phase 1 and phase 2 happens so quickly that the intermediate compounds don't spill out. If the liver doesn't get this support, however, phase 2 is compromised. The partly transformed toxins spill out of the liver, return to circulation in the blood and lymph, and travel back to the tissues and cells, where they cause damage. The other organs of detoxification might try to compensate, but none can do what the liver can do. A cascade of stresses on different systems can set in, which strains the body more. Knowing this, you can begin to see why fasting on its own, even though it helps accelerate the release of toxins from tissues, might be harmful to health. There are no nutrients coming in to help with the processing and neutralizing stage that must occur next.

THE SPECTRUM OF CLEANSING

This basic understanding of the mechanics of detoxification helps explain why different detox programs have different effects and results. Some are designed to release toxins in a rush, others, to let them out slowly. But they vary in how successfully they "equalize" the intensity of detox mode and the intensity of liver detoxification, and this determines, to my mind, their safety for the average person. With this in mind, here's a guide to the most popular detox programs of the moment, and where Clean lies in relation to them.

Water Fasting

Water fasting is the most intense form of detoxification, and has been used by spiritual leaders, including Jesus and the Buddha. Since only water is consumed, once the signal to enter detox mode is triggered, tissues release toxins and mucus into circulation—and don't stop. In fact, the release gets more intense as the days go by. In ancient times, when this method was used primarily for spiritual reasons, there were no chemicals in the environment and so there were far fewer accumulated toxins to be released back into circulation. With our level of toxicity today and our nutrient-deficient bodies, water fasting can be dangerous. More toxicity is released, with a lot less nutrient support for liver detoxification.

I have witnessed many people try this method over the years. They all got very weak and sleepy and could not go for long, with the exception of one individual who had been cleansing consistently for twenty-five years and lived a very clean life in between detox programs. Although a few water fasters had no other problems but fatigue, many others suffered nausea, headaches, vomiting, diarrhea, skin rashes, and other symptoms. Though I didn't personally witness the more severe cases, they occurred and, tragically, included one death, that of a man who tried this fast to cure his cancer. (It is impossible to say what killed him, the fasting, the cancer, or a combination of both.) Nevertheless, I have also seen, heard of, and read of people healing themselves from apparently "incurable" diseases using this intense and controversial fasting method.

The Master Cleanse
The Master Cleanse is a liquid-only detox program that has recently gained popularity. You drink only

water with lemon, grade-B maple syrup, and cayenne pepper for as long as you can handle it. It is generally well tolerated, but as with the water fasting, I have witnessed cases where it went very wrong. Even if well tolerated, the Master Cleanse is more beneficial to those who undertake a cleanse for emotional, mental, and maybe spiritual reasons than for the physical benefits. Once toxins and mucus are released into the blood, they must be eliminated from the body, and the Master Cleanse method enhances elimination only by the irritation that cayenne pepper causes on the intestinal mucosa, not by "binding" fiber to the toxins to prevent reabsorption and pulling them out. The main reason the Master Cleanse is incomplete is because it does not accomplish what I consider to be the most important aspect of a detox program in our modern world: the restoration of the intestinal flora and the integrity of the intestinal wall.

Juice Fasting

In a juice fast you consume nothing but freshly made vegetable and fruit juices and water or herbal teas. This slows down the detox intensity seen in water fasting, although not by too much, so detoxification is still quite intense. The juices provide the nutrients needed for both phases of liver detoxification—they need to be primarily green (vegetable) juices with few of the sweet fruit juices. Kale is considered the king of juicing vegetables.

However, you still need a good knowledge of nutrients to create and benefit from a juice fast. You need to add minerals via supplements, and good fiber or herbal laxatives are essential as there is no fiber in the juices. Though hunger tends to diminish naturally, most people report that a juice fast works best when they are able to take a sabbatical from regular demands of life at a retreat center—if only because it takes strong discipline to avoid the temptations of food. This type of cleanse also fails to rebuild the intestinal flora and therefore is not complete, unless you add in a side program of herbal antimicrobials and probiotics.

Blended Fasting

Blended fasting involves pureeing instead of juicing your vegetables and fruits, so that their fiber makes you fuller, and may add emollients like avocado or olive oil to increase fat quantity. This slows down toxin release as it takes more energy to digest, but the advantage of this method is that you are less hungry, and the fiber that remains in the drinks sequesters (grabs) the toxins in the intestinal lumen and carries them out, preventing them from being reabsorbed into the bloodstream. As a detox program, it is of medium-high intensity. For this reason, blended smoothies and shakes are an integral part of the Clean program.

Raw Food

A raw-food diet is usually seen more as a lifestyle diet than as a cleanse, but I use it as a detox tool for some patients, because it combines the benefits of the juice and blended fasts with a little more solidity in the daily diet in the form of raw-food meals. As raw-food devotees will confirm, the power of enzyme-rich raw foods both aids the release of toxicity and supports the liver in its processing. The downside is that for many people living busy city lives, it is hard to shop for and prepare.

Nutritional Cleanses

Nutritional cleanses are a recent addition to the detox world. You drink shakes that have been specially designed to deliver protein, fat, and some carbohydrate in liquid form along with all the nutrients, antioxidants, vitamins, and minerals needed by the liver. You also eat a reduced number of solid-food meals that will not irritate or tax your system. This kind of cleanse is often done using so-called medical foods—powdered protein shakes made with natural ingredients and an array of natural supplements. Over several weeks, toxins are released consistently with all the necessary support to neutralize them successfully. A huge benefit of this modern method is that it provides protein, which can attract some of the circulating toxins, thereby preventing them from reentering the tissues. (This is especially important to know should you go on to do a specialized heavy-metal cleanse; heavy metals bind to proteins, which help prevent them from circulating to their favored locations, such as the brain.) The Clean program is a type of nutritional cleanse.

Ayurvedic Detoxification Programs

Ayurvedic detoxification programs are slower in their toxic release than many other cleansing routines, because they use cooked foods, yet slow does not mean ineffective. Many conditions are better addressed by longer-term, lower-intensity detoxification methods. Furthermore, the ancient *panchakarma* techniques get many of their great results from taking into consideration your individual constitution (the *kapha, vata, pitta* body types mentioned in the "Quantum Toxins" section of chapter 5).

The Elimination Diet

The Elimination Diet depends on eliminating foods that are hard to digest or cause allergic reactions.

It can be used on its own as a detox program. When you eliminate hard-to-digest foods and eat mainly organic vegetables, brown rice, beans, fish or lean protein, fruits, and nuts, you free up much of the energy wasted on initiating and sustaining immune responses. This alone can greatly clear up many people's symptoms, although it takes longer than more targeted cleanses.

WHY CLEAN?

There is no one single "right" method for building and maintaining balanced health. The range of tools available for promoting detoxification is impressive, and, with experience and guidance and attention to some disclaimers, you can use all the methods at varying points in your life. Extensive experience with all of them has shown me that the largest number of people get the greatest results from a nutritional cleanse. Bringing about an ongoing release of toxicity backed by a steady supply of nourishment, they achieve in a relatively short time (three weeks) the kind of results that the more challenging juice fasts might achieve in seven to ten days. The Clean program that you will follow in this book uses the principles of the nutritional cleanse to create a detox program you can easily do at home, with freshly made foods and drinks. (A medical-foods version of it is also available in a kit from www.the cleanprogram.com.) It is safe and practical and has been tested extensively on hundreds of patients under my medical supervision.

To design Clean, I drew on the extensive research and knowledge of Functional Medicine, a model of healing that exemplifies the integration of Western, evidence-based science with an Eastern, holistic approach to deliver individualized care that truly gets to the root of disease. Functional Medicine is "open-minded" medicine in action, benefiting from ancient health knowledge while using the most advanced technology when necessary.

GETTING STARTED

Clean is custom-built to incorporate the five essential functions of detoxification.

1. Reduce the workload of digestion. The small daily loss of energy funds to allergy responses, even if you don't overtly feel them happening, is taking its energy toll and contributing to the "dullness" that most of us experience day in and day out. Consum-

ing less solid food and leaving out irritants lead to a reallocation of energy to the processes of detoxification.

2. Restore the twelve-hour window. After the signal to enter detox mode starts, around eight hours after your last meal, the typical modern body needs about four hours to do a deep cleaning. Few of us get this today, because we snack and drink until late at night.

3. Rebuild the inner environment. Acidity is lowered, the intestinal flora is rebalanced in favor of the beneficial bacteria, and the intestinal wall gets a chance to heal. Creating this balanced and stable environment reduces cravings for the foods that cause toxicity, which supports long-term maintenance of a clean state.

4. Support the liver. Nutrients are delivered that ensure that the liver can perform phase 1 and 2 functions efficiently, keeping you safe.

5. Enhance elimination. Once toxins are released and neutralized, they must be discarded along with their mucus coating. Clean incorporates supplements and techniques to ensure that this happens effectively.

Clean preparation is done in three steps:

Step 1. Preparing Your Mind: Easing into the Program
Step 2. Preparing Your Life: Schedule and Home
Step 3. Preparing Your Body: Eliminating Irritants

You do not have to wait until toxicity is eliminated across the planet—it may be too late. You do not have to settle for symptom control and its dangers.

You do not have to give up on your search for a powerful way to repair the damage of living in our toxic world.

You are about to experience what happens when your body is given back the magic abilities it was born with.

The Clean program is your guide.

People of all walks of life have done it successfully.

So can you. Get Clean!

Clean works best when you complete the full three weeks, but the program will also yield results after one or two weeks. Some of my patients build up to the complete three-week program, while others jump in and complete the whole Clean program the first time out. Wherever you are in this spectrum, it is important to remember that every change you make is an important one.

Please read through the following section, which describes the whole program, before starting, as it contains information that will help you plan, accomplish, and benefit from Clean in the most successful way.

BEFORE YOU START CLEAN

People with certain conditions should not cleanse or detox. Please do not proceed if any of these apply to you at the moment:

- You are pregnant or breastfeeding.
- You have type 1 (insulin-dependent) diabetes.
- You are currently living with advanced cancer and are losing weight rapidly.
- You are taking a medication that needs a stable blood concentration, including medication for preventing blood clots (such as Coumadin), antiarrhythmics (such as Tikosyn), or anticonvulsants (such as Tegretol). Stable blood concentrations of drugs may get disrupted as absorption rates change, leaving you on too high or too low a dose. Consult with your doctor and do not proceed on any kind of detoxification program without supervision of an expert.

• You are currently living with any other disease that needs close monitoring and in which slight changes in your body chemistry could pose a threat.

ARE YOU SPENT?

There is another group of people who should not start the Clean or any other detox program. These are people who present with a clinical picture that is not recognized by most traditional physicians, but has been identified and treated extensively by my colleague, Dr. Frank Lipman. He has named this the "Spent" syndrome, and it refers to patients who are exhausted and have low blood pressure and a host of other symptoms attributable to the depletion of their hypothalamic-pituitary-adrenal axis, the body's stress-regulating system.

Depletion of the adrenal system, the "Spent" condition, is rarely diagnosed by conventional doctors, largely because most blood tests and other laboratory evaluations come back as normal, despite the patients' experience of being constantly exhausted. This means they continue on without treatment as stress takes its toll on the body, when replenishing the adrenal function holistically is actually what is indicated. Dr. Lipman, my partner at the Eleven Eleven Wellness Center in

New York, and I are seeing that this condition disproportionately affects women. This could be because their hormonal systems are more complex, because they tend to express the effects of fatigue more acutely, or because women, as natural caregivers, are more likely to let themselves reach a point of burnout before asking for help. But the condition does not discriminate between the sexes and it's likely that all of us, women and men, go "Spent" at times in our lives.

Your answers to the following questions will help determine whether you have a problem with your adrenal function:

- Does it take you longer than average to recover from illnesses or injuries?
- Do you regularly have difficulty getting out of bed in the morning?
- Do you feel a sense of ongoing fatigue that is not relieved by a good night's sleep?
- Do you feel light-headed when getting up from a lying-down position?
- Do you have abnormally low blood pressure?
- Do you have extreme sensitivity to cold or tend to feel cold in environments where others do not?
- Do you have a chronic level of anxiety or have you ever had panic attacks?

- Do you have periods of depression or frequent crying jags (also a hallmark of toxicity)?
- Do you have a tendency to bruise easily?

Although some of these symptoms are similar to those of toxicity, as a group they are more specific to the adrenal weakness the Spent program is designed to help. If you answered yes to two or more of these questions, it is important to find a health-care practitioner who understands how to check your level of adrenal function and work with you to improve it. Embarking on a detox program would be counterproductive and even harmful if you are Spent, as you will not have necessary energy to support the detox and intestinal rebuilding processes. Once you have rested and reactivated your adrenal glands, a detox program will be in order.

I highly recommend that you read Dr. Lipman's book, *Spent*, which describes the syndrome and its treatment plan in detail. The ability to tune in to what you need and distinguish between the conditions of toxicity and of being Spent may be one of the most important tools you can use to create a future free of hospital visits and prescription drugs—and full of vibrant health.

If you have any ongoing health problems whatsoever, please consult your doctor before engaging in any detox program, including Clean. If your doctor does not support you or does not give you well-explained, sound reasons why you should not begin a program, I recommend you change doctors and consider working with a professional familiar with Functional Medicine, who is trained in the ways that sickness and disease can have roots in toxicity and a weakened ability to detoxify. You will learn more about working with a wellness partner in chapter 8, "After the Cleanse."

STEP 1. PREPARING YOUR MIND: EASING INTO THE PROGRAM

Anytime you take on a project to improve an aspect of your life, you spend a little time planning and preparing for it. The Clean program is no different. Although it is a simple program to follow once you are started, it will require you to change some habits for a few weeks, and that can sometimes be challenging. If you take some time to prepare your mind, your schedule, and home—and, most important, your body— before you start, you will maximize your chances of success.

Gabriella came to my office after a number of different gastroenterologists had failed to help her improve her condition. She was diagnosed as having "ulcerative colitis," an autoimmune problem. She had two young kids and no help. Her greatest problem was that she had an urgent need to stop wherever she found a restroom. Her breaking point had come the previous week, when she found herself at a Seven-Eleven, unable to leave the bathroom, with two toddlers inside the bathroom with her. I instructed her to start Clean.

A week later she came for a follow-up visit and told me she wanted to stop. Her problem was that even though she was feeling better, it was time-consuming to prepare blended foods for herself. Her "urgency" feelings had almost completely gone away, but she seemed to have forgotten how much time she had spent the previous week in public restrooms. I reminded her of our previous conversation in detail, when she had come to me and described her problem and frustration with her doctors. As she herself started vividly remembering, I saw in her face the unmistakable expression of an "Aha!" moment. We never talked again about the time needed for preparing healthy food. She completed three weeks without a complaint. She still follows the Elimination Diet and continues to fine-tune her lifestyle to support vibrant health.

Thinking of the big picture puts everything into perspective, giving you strength to sustain a change in behavior. This is also true on the flip side—if you fail to follow through with a plan you decided to complete. Judging or punishing yourself will not help. Guilt is as toxic as emotions come. If you find yourself failing, you can look at it as an opportunity to learn how to detoxify guilt itself. I have seen many people transformed by the initial shock of guilt, once they acquire the ability to put that force to work for them. It's an emotional judo of sorts: the defender redirects the attacker's charge to the defender's own advantage. Transformation is happening all the time. Failing is just proof that you are trying. Practice makes perfect. One day at a time. The right mental attitude is integral to completing this program and transforming your health.

One of the first patients I guided through the Clean program was my friend Moshe. He listened very carefully to my instructions and then, with a serious face, said, "Alex, I have a big problem. I won't be able to do this."

"Why not?" I asked him.

"I really, really like bread," he responded.

I told him what I have since told hundreds of patients. Do not think of Clean as something you will be doing for the rest of your life, as changing your diet and lifestyle for good. That's an overwhelming and, frankly, undesirable prospect for most people. Rather, think of it as an experiment. If you're like 90 percent of the population, you have probably eaten, drunk, and lived guided by your free will for most of your life, and knowing that you can return to free will after this experiment will reduce the stress of a long-term commitment. Yet I can almost guarantee there will be a natural shift as a result of doing Clean. You may just find that after you complete the program, you will look at food differently. You may simply not *want* to go back to what you were doing and eating before. You may want to make new choices. This is different from not being *allowed* to.

Like everything in life worth working for, this program will take commitment and discipline. The first three days may be hard, but most people soon adjust to the restriction in food choices and quantity. Within a week, they say they can't understand how they ate so much before. Often they realize with surprise how much their life revolves around food. A detox program can offer a new perspective on what the body actually needs to function well—and how much our tendency to excess is more suffocating than supportive.

In my experience, people who complete the program *are* changed by the end of it. They have a new attitude toward food and a different experience of it. A resetting

Nature Versus Nurture

Eating three meals a day every day is a fairly recent cultural invention in the span of human history. For millennia, our genes evolved in a world where feast or famine was the norm, so our bodies adapted over generations to be able to store excess food whenever it was found, to fuel us through periods when food was scarce. The industrialization of food in the last hundred and fifty years has made "excess" the new norm, yet our genes can't adapt that quickly. They still eagerly store whenever they get the chance—which in modern life is all the time. This disconnect between genetic design inside and rapid change outside is the root of much of the conflicts we feel about eating.

of their taste buds has occurred, which makes them desire healthier and more natural foods. This is very different from knowing that healthier foods are good for you, but having to force yourself to consume them. It is the "You eat what you are" phenomenon in action.

For Moshe and many others, before they did Clean, certain foods that contributed to the toxic, tired state, such as bread and sugar, were almost magnetically appealing, keeping them stuck in a cycle. But after losing the chemicals and additives and getting a break from sugars, simple carbs, and stimulants, they had so changed their inner environment that they lost the cravings for their old favorites. Their senses, cleared of chemicals and sugars, found more to enjoy in fresh foods; they could "hear" the way their bodies responded to real food over junk food. Suddenly, bright green broccoli gave the delight that only used to come from Rocky Road ice cream. Improving the environment inside the body is much more effective for "cleaning up" poor eating habits than using sheer willpower or the power of positive thinking alone. It's a universal truth: when you are fit and healthy, you crave the good-quality foods that maintain that state.

If your instinct is pushing you toward a detoxification program but you need motivation, just look around at people on the street, or in the mall, or in the airport. How healthy and happy does the average person look? Read some of the health Web sites that are talking honestly about the real state of health in America today. Too many people are sick. Too many people are taking medications, going to the doctor, or suffering with some kind of symptom. Half of Americans will have heart disease or cancer in their lives. The other half will likely develop other kinds of conditions and diseases that will continue to make the pharmaceutical industry one of the most profitable industries of all time. So as you consider whether you can successfully do the Clean program, it can be helpful to ask yourself, do you want to be a number in the American bad-health statistics? If you do what most Americans do and you eat what most Americans eat, how can you expect a different outcome?

I met Frank, a forty-year-old New Yorker, six months after he'd undergone emergency abdominal surgery to remove his gallbladder. Though he was a little heavy and his skin looked dull and puffy, his surgeon and his specialist had declared him fixed. But he didn't feel it. He had been suffering from mysterious abdominal pains since the surgery and he lived in a constant state of anxiety that the pain was a message telling him a tumor was waiting to get him. Since nobody had advised him otherwise, he continued to eat his lifelong diet consisting of large amounts of meat, fatty treats, dairy foods, and alcohol. These things filled up his anxious stomach, comforted his mind, and relaxed his emotions temporarily.

After doing a full physical evaluation, I was confident that Frank had a strong constitution and had generally recovered well from his surgery, but the symptoms he reported were signs that his intestinal flora was severely altered. His starchy, sweet diet, in combination with the antibiotics, anesthetics, and painkillers from the surgery had devastated his good bacteria. All these toxins had created dysbiosis and now the yeast that had overgrown in the intestines were releasing toxins causing abdominal bloating and pain. Worse, they were making him crave more sugary, starchy foods.

Frank was amazed at how, after completing the Clean program, his energy returned, his mood was elevated, and the pains began to disappear. When he reintroduced the old foods back into his diet—caffeine, red meats, fatty foods, dairy products, and more than one or two alcoholic drinks a week—he discovered that they irritated his digestive system and caused abdominal pains. The less he consumed these things, the less pain he felt. He had misinterpreted the earlier "message" from his body: the pain was not an omen of a tumor; it was a distress signal from an intestinal tract that was irritated and inflamed. The great benefit of his cleanse was the end of these cravings—and a new confidence in the strength of his health. As he cleaned out this debris, Frank began to hear something new: his body was hungry for different kinds of things. Instead of comforting, heavy foods, he wanted fresh vegetables and other foods that made him feel clear and sharp. He made smoothies with protein powder and went to the gym instead of having a cup of coffee. He told me, "I finally feel like I am listening to my body and I get it: I am what I eat—and I eat what I am!"

STEP 2. PREPARING YOUR LIFE: SCHEDULE AND HOME

In some ways doing the Clean program at home is more convenient than retreating to a fasting center or spa for a cleanse, but it has its challenges. Changes of habit are hard for everyone to accomplish, no matter what level of diet and lifestyle they're starting from, and changes in eating and drinking are some of the hardest. When we attempt to break free of them, we get moody and irritable or start craving the things we are trying to quit. Even though the Clean program addresses these issues nutritionally and biochemically, you have to be your own main support team. If you set up a schedule and system in advance, you will maximize your chances of success.

Put Clean on Your Schedule

Like anything worth investing effort and energy in, you have to make time for Clean. Plenty of busy people, from parents to business executives, from students to entertainers, have finished the program. They'll all agree that getting three weeks free of obligations or social events is a fantasy, so don't wait for months to start. Waiting for the perfect window of quiet time probably means you'll never do it. What you can do, however, is plan the program for a period with minimal travel and start on a weekend if the week tends to involve business and social events. This will give you time to get used to the new menu and go through the first few days of adjustment outside of the workplace. Also note that too many changes at the same time can be hard to sustain, so try to start your program at a time when you are not moving, changing jobs, divorcing, or going through other major changes. (But some people do best during times of total change—you may be one of them.)

When you have decided on a start date, put it in your calendar just as you would any other commitment, such as a trip or work project. Note the dates you will start the Elimination Diet preparation phase and mark out Week 1, Week 2, and Week 3. Weekly planner charts are provided for you in the next section of the book, but it helps to put some of the optional activities, from exercise to massage, right onto whatever calendar you look at daily. You will also need to make some time for shopping for all the ingredients you plan to use each week. Block out times for this each week; finding your fridge empty halfway through the week is an unnecessary obstacle.

Once you are in the swing of the program, it's fairly easy to follow your normal lifestyle. Make the choice to do things differently and stay away from the cocktail hour and meals with friends and family for a few days. You might even take your dinnertime liquid-meal jar to a friend's house.

Setting Up Your Kitchen

Getting a system set up for Clean that is both functional and supportive is very important. The anchor of this system is the kitchen. Millions of people today rarely cook—they eat out for most of their meals. Their challenge will be to *use* the kitchen and to find the time to organize and prepare foods daily. For others, the kitchen is the hub of a busy home. Their challenge may come from the tempting foods it is stocked with for other members of the family. If you are the household chef, determine how far you can go in disrupting the status quo. A personal commitment to your own goals might be the only thing that helps you get through preparing other peoples' meals as you sip your vegetable juice. Know that after the first week this will get easier. But also remember that anything you do for yourself will help the whole family. It's not too much to ask others to adapt slightly to accommodate you from time to time.

Take a few minutes to look in all your kitchen drawers and cabinets. See how many packaged products you have. What food do you have in boxes, jars, bags, tubes, and cans? Read the ingredients, familiarize yourself with what you were eating before, and then throw away or give away whatever is counter to the way you want to eat now. This should include anything that is going to tempt you to stray from your Clean meals and snacks.

You will need three basic essentials to complete the program that will all be important for maintaining the benefits over the long term. Although the best versions of them can be expensive, you can find affordable ones that will work fine. Since they'll help you long after Clean is finished, they should be seen as an investment in your well-being.

1. A blender. Smoothies and soups are a very important part of the Clean program. I recommend a high-speed blender such as Vitamix, but any good blender with a powerful motor will do. Some recipes also call for a food processor for solid ingredients.

2. A juicer. There are lots of good juicers on the market today. My favorite brand is Breville, which makes powerful and easy-to-clean products.

3. A source of pure water. Anyone on the path to being Clean needs to use pure water. Tap water today carries too many chemicals to support you as

you actively detoxify. Though it's possible to buy bottled water during the program or use a bottled-water delivery system, these options are expensive over time and damaging to the environment. Jug filters will take chlorine out of the water, but leave many of the harmful substances. Your Clean program is a good time to invest in a water filtration system for your kitchen sink. A reverse osmosis filtration system lets you wash foods in clean water, drink clean water, and use it for your Clean program soups and smoothies. These are available starting for around $300 and increase in price as they get more effective. My preferred source is listed in the "Staying Clean" section of chapter 8. Whatever you decide on, try to use the purest water possible during the program.

Prepare a few clean jars and food-grade plastic containers so you are equipped to take your liquid meals and your daily lunches with you to work and elsewhere.

After familiarizing yourself with the ingredients needed for the meals and smoothies, juices, and soups, investigate where you can buy the healthiest ingredients possible, like a local farmers' market, health-food store, or a supermarket with a good organic selection. In addition to buying what you need for Clean, remember to buy the foods that will help you when you feel cravings, such as raw nuts and herbal teas.

STEP 3. PREPARING YOUR BODY: ELIMINATING IRRITANTS

When it comes to cleaning, detoxifying, and restoring the body, it's not ideal to go from zero to sixty overnight. There is some groundwork to be done. A few days of doing the Elimination Diet before you begin Clean will ease your body into the program, by clearing out of your body foods and chemicals you may be allergic or sensitive to and freeing up energy for detoxification.

Reduce Your Exposure to Toxins

Reduce your exposure to toxins in your environment and in your diet.

TOXINS IN YOUR ENVIRONMENT

The following are common everyday sources of toxicity: car exhaust, gardening and lawn chemicals, dry-cleaning products, heating systems, air-conditioning systems (use hepa filters), chlorine in swimming pools, mattresses containing fire retardants, lead paint, cleaning products and waxes, aluminum-containing deodorant, fluoride-containing toothpaste, cosmetics, pots and pans whose cooking surfaces are coated with aluminum or Teflon, electromagnetic radiation from electronics, and cell phones.

As you set up your kitchen, notice where in your home and work environments you are exposed to unnecessary toxins. The most obvious category will be your household cleaning supplies. Read their labels just as you did with food. When you go grocery shopping for Clean, pick up one or two toxin-free home cleaners to try, so that you start the process of lowering your toxic load in addition to cleaning out your diet. Over the coming weeks, begin to notice where and when you are exposed to some of the most common daily toxins. Your kitchen, your bathroom, and your garage as well as your work environment will likely contain a considerable number of toxic products. Avoid what you can, replace the products you can, and consider how to lower your daily exposure. There is a plethora of information online about making your home and life toxin-free and it can happen in small steps (see "Clean Resources" in the appendix for further information).

TOXINS IN YOUR DIET

The duration of this preparation phase will vary, depending on the characteristics of your existing diet

228 • ALEJANDRO JUNGER, M.D.

and lifestyle. The cleaner you are to begin with, the shorter amount of time you can spend on preparation.

- Three to four days of the Elimination Diet is enough if you have done some cleansing programs recently or follow a whole-food-based diet with minimal meat, milk products, and wheat and almost no packaged, canned, or fast foods.
- One week is enough if you consider yourself an average eater, with a diet that typically contains some or all of the following: packaged foods, red meat, baked goods, dairy products, sugar products, caffeine, alcohol. One week is the average amount of time people spend on the Elimination Diet before starting the Clean program.
- Follow the Elimination Diet for two weeks before starting Clean if your diet includes a lot of fast food, boxed or packaged foods, sodas, junk food, and alcohol. If you have the time, you will get maximum benefit from Clean when you start it.

This preparation step will minimize withdrawals from caffeine and other chemicals in foods that can be a cause of headaches, nausea, and all kinds of other annoying symptoms during a detox program. It will also help blunt a possible "healing crisis": sometimes a body that has been dulled with processed foods and deprived of nutrients responds in a dramatic way to eliminating toxins and obtaining adequate nutrients. The immune and repair systems can suddenly bounce back into full working mode and unsettle things on the surface, causing skin breakouts, fevers, and an array of symptoms that make you feel as if you are falling ill, when in fact they are signs of the body's waking up and getting back in the game. Though a healing crisis is ultimately a good thing, it will disrupt your life and can be uncomfortable or even alarming. If you prepare by following the basic Elimination Diet for a few days you will avoid any of these problems.

The foods you eat in this phase are also the main ingredients in your Clean food and liquid meals. After this preparation, you will feel lighter in the body, sharper in the mind, and confident that you have the adaptability and motivation to accomplish the Clean program in full.

FAQs: Smoking and Prescription Medication

Q: I smoke. Do I have to cut this out too?

A: Smokers have different experiences than nonsmokers do during Clean. Some use it as a chance to quit cold turkey. Others find that smoking starts to lose its appeal as their palate and sensitivity to toxins opens up. At the very least, many naturally become more mindful of each cigarette, just as they are becoming more mindful of food. Even if you make no changes in your cigarette consumption, go ahead and do the whole program, knowing you are boosting your detoxification ability and creating a "clean canvas" in your body where you may just start to feel the effects of cigarettes in a different way. Smoking affects detoxification by accelerating phase 1 in the liver and it will detract from your achieving the best results.

Q: I am taking prescription medication prescribed by my doctor. Should I stop taking it?

A: If you are taking any kind of prescription drug, do not stop taking it during this program. Many prescription drugs can be safely stopped, but some cannot. Certain serious conditions require a consistent level of medication in the blood. Any change in diet can cause a change in the medication's absorption rate, which can result in a higher or lower concentration in the blood. In the case of blood thinners, antiarrhythmic drugs, antiepileptic drugs, and chemotherapy agents, this can be life-threatening.

Eating from the Elimination Diet

Eat breakfast, lunch, and dinner at your regular times, choosing only foods and drinks from the "Yes" side and excluding all foods from the "No" side of the "Include/Exclude List" below. Since the "Yes" side of the list almost certainly does not contain some foods that you consume daily, you will need to make substitutions. Start using some of the recipes for the Clean program now (see chapter 11, "The Clean Recipes"). They are all Elimination Diet recipes, so they do the thinking for you.

Breakfast is the hardest meal to change, because bread, cereal, milk, and eggs are not allowed. Try a liquid breakfast like the Energy Smoothie with Almond Butter and Cardamom. You could also eat fish, chicken, or vegetables from the previous evening's meal; make a bowl of brown rice or quinoa "cereal" with some fruit and nuts or have some almond butter on fruit.

For lunch, eat salads containing the permitted protein types, soups, or other dishes using beans, lentils, and permitted grains, instead of sandwiches, wraps, and burritos or other typical meals.

For dinner use some of the Clean recipes here as guidelines and add green vegetables and quinoa instead of white rice, pasta, or potatoes. Steamed fish, grilled chicken, and baked or roasted vegetables are common meals during this phase.

Note that this is the time to begin decreasing your caffeine use. You may drink green tea if you need it and you can also try yerba mate, which has a stimulating effect similar to that of coffee. The more you can avoid caffeine, however, the better. In general, drink plenty of pure water during this preparation phase. You can add lemon, cucumber, and mint to it to make it more interesting. Herbal teas help substitute for black tea and coffee but need to be taken in addition to plenty of plain water, not instead of it.

Buy organic products whenever possible. These few weeks of preparing for and doing the Clean program are an opportunity to significantly reduce the toxic load in the body. Reducing exposure to toxins in your food is a no-brainer if you have access to and can afford organic produce. The most important thing to spend money on are organic animal products, because toxins accumulate as they go up the food chain. Look for organic, hormone-free chicken and meat and choose wild fish over farmed fish. When buying plant foods, spend money on organic fruits such as peaches, apples, and berries, and organic vegetables such as celery, spinach, carrots, cucumbers, and beans before worrying about thick-skinned produce like avocadoes and squash. Do the best that you and your wallet can, and always wash your produce very well.

Remove the Obstacles, Add What's Missing

Eating according to the Elimination Diet will achieve the following important detox goals:

1. Remove from your diet the packaged and processed foods and drinks that contain additives, preservatives, and other chemicals, including "hidden sources" you might not think about, such as condiments and sauces.

2. Reduce potential irritants and allergens in the diet. Some of the most common foods in the American diet have hidden irritating effects. The nightshade family of vegetables—tomatoes, sweet peppers, eggplants, and potatoes—can cause sensitivity. In Ayurvedic thinking they cause the buildup of *amma* in some body types when eaten in excess, suppressing digestive strength. Strawberries, chocolate, shellfish, and certain nuts are also common allergens.

3. Reduce acidity and create a more alkaline inner environment. Red meat, milk products, bananas, and excessive grains such as wheat are all acid-making foods. These are also the main "mucus-making"

YES Include These Foods	NO Exclude These Foods
Fruits: whole fruits, un-sweetened, frozen or water-packed, diluted natural juices	Oranges, orange juice, grapefruit, strawberries, grapes, banana
Dairy Substitutes: rice, oat and nut milks such as almond milk and coconut milk	Dairy and eggs, milk, cheese, cottage cheese, cream, yogurt, butter, ice cream, nondairy creamers
Non-gluten Grains and Starch: brown rice, millet, quinoa, amaranth, buckwheat	Wheat, corn, barley, spelt, kamut, rye, couscous, oats
Animal Protein: cold water fish, wild game, lean lamb, duck, chicken, turkey	Raw fish, pork, beef, veal, sausage, cold cuts, canned meats, hot dogs, shellfish
Vegetable Protein: split peas, lentils, legumes	Soybean products (soy sauce, soybean oil in processed foods, tempeh, tofu, soy milk, soy yogurt)
Nuts and Seeds: sesame, pumpkin, and sunflower seeds; hazelnuts; pecans; almonds; cashews; walnuts	Peanuts, peanut butter, pistachios, macadamia nuts

YES Include These Foods	NO Exclude These Foods
Vegetables: preferably fresh, raw, steamed, sautéed, juiced, roasted	Corn, creamed vegetables, tomatoes, potatoes, eggplants, peppers
Oils: cold pressed olive, flax, safflower, sesame, almond, sunflower, canola, pumpkin, walnut	Butter, margarine, shortening, processed oils, salad dressings, mayonnaise, spreads
Drinks: filtered or distilled water, green tea, herbal teas, seltzer or mineral water, yerba mate	Alcohol, coffee, caffeinated beverages, soda pop, soft drinks
Sweeteners: brown rice syrup, agave syrup, stevia	Refined sugar, white or brown sugars, honey, maple syrup, high-fructose corn syrup, evaporated cane juice
Condiments: vinegar, all spices, sea salt, pepper, basil, carob, cinnamon, cumin, dill, garlic, ginger, mustard, oregano, parsley, rosemary, turmeric, thyme	Chocolate, ketchup, relish, chutney, soy sauce, barbecue sauce, teriyaki sauce, other similar condiments

foods that cause the stickiness in the intestines that is counter to healthy nutrient absorption and elimination. During and after Clean, the more you can avoid acidifying foods and fill the diet with alkalinizing ones, the better.

4. Remove foods that have an inflammatory effect in the body. Simple carbohydrates such as sugars and grains, especially refined grains (white flour, white rice), cause the body to release greater amounts of insulin into the blood to regulate absorption of the sugars into the cells. Insulin is a pro-inflammatory hormone. The hydrogenated cooking oils known as "trans fats" also cause inflammation. (Cold-pressed oils are not hydrogenated.)

5. Fill the diet with anti-inflammatory nutrients: omega-3 fatty acids from fish; polyphenols (plant-based compounds) from berries; and many plant-based compounds that boost liver detoxification.

6. Remove foods, such as grapefruits, that tend to suppress certain reactions in the liver detoxification function.

7. Remove foods that tend to have fungi on them (peanuts) or that feed the yeast in the intestines causing dysbiosis (sugars, alcohol, and dairy products). Remember, alcohol is made by fermenting grain or fruit sugars into ethanol. Its yeasty mix contributes to dys-

biosis. It also contains its own mix of preservatives (sulfites in wine) and is a depressant.

8. Remove caffeine, alcohol, and, ideally, cigarettes, all of which tax the adrenal glands, negatively impact liver detoxification, and create free radicals that can damage cells (especially DNA and RNA), particularly when used daily and in quantity.

9. Remove the most pesticide-laden crops and hormone- and antibiotic-filled meat, dairy, and egg products. Also remove the main sources of genetically modified foods that go unlabeled into our food supply, the damaging effects of which we are still learning about (especially in the soy, corn, and wheat supply stream).

The pH Factor

Some foods actually contain acids or alkalis (soluble salts) and other foods create acidity or alkalinity in the body when combined with juices and digestive acids (acidic lemons have an alkalinizing influence). As mentioned earlier, a diet rich in alkali-forming foods is a key to ongoing good health. It helps with detoxification, as the body is already working to eliminate the acidic waste products of metabolism—you don't want to add to the burden. The desired state within the body is slightly more alkaline than neutral. You can easily check your

Acid-Forming Foods

Alcohol
Bananas
Beans (most kinds)
Beef
Chicken
Corn
Dairy products
Eggs
Fish
Grains
Lamb
Nuts
Pork
Plums & Prunes
Rice
Sodas
Shell fish
Sugar
Sweet potatoes
Tomatoes (processed)
Turkey
Unripe fruit

Alkali-Forming Foods

Most ripe fruits
Most vegetables
Barley
Buckwheat
Soy beans
Lima beans
Azuki beans
Brazil nuts
Sprouted almonds
Honey
Millet

own pH state by using litmus paper strips to test your saliva. They are available at vitamin stores.

A very basic guide to common acidifying and alkalinizing foods can be found on the next page.

The health implications of our acidic lives is currently being seen in the loss of bone density. More and more women are being diagnosed with osteopenia or osteoporosis. Most doctors prescribe supplemental calcium for this and instruct their patients to consume more dairy products to get "bone-building" calcium. What is not understood is that the bone is like an Alka-Seltzer tablet and will fizzle and release its salts in an attempt to alkalinize blood that has become chronically acid. The bones are dissolving because the blood is already acidic—and then dairy, an acid-forming food, is prescribed as a treatment. Moreover, calcium is not deposited in the bones without adequate levels of vitamin D, yet a test of vitamin D levels is rarely ordered by primary-care physicians. If a diagnosis of toxicity and testing for overly acidic conditions were the first response, a life-building, not life-harming, protocol could be advised, which could help the body reverse its harmful course.

Eating Out During the Elimination Diet

It is not hard to eat outside the home while you are on the Elimination Diet. You will have to make smart choices about where you go—and then spend a moment with the menu before choosing. A pizza and pasta restaurant will make it harder, though not impossible, to avoid the "no" foods.

Some of the common restaurant meals that will not fit the Elimination Diet requirements include sandwiches, hamburgers, pizza, wheat pasta, sushi, tomato-based sauces, tofu dishes, wheat-noodle dishes, anything with Asian soy sauces, baked potatoes, omelettes and egg-based breakfasts, wheat and corn tortillas, burritos, empanadas, lattes, cappuccinos, all coffee drinks, and desserts of all kinds unless they are fruit salad or plain fruit.

There are still plenty of options to choose from when you go out. Pick a meal on the menu that has protein, vegetables, and a permitted grain such as brown rice. (Indian restaurants, with their wide array of vegetarian foods and lentil and bean dishes, are a good bet.) Just ask the waiter to take your wine glass away and not bring the bread basket, naan bread, or corn chips, and you will find this way of eating much easier than you might have imagined.

Marco, a native of Italy, came to see me a few days after he had been diagnosed with advanced lung cancer. His cancer had already spread (metastasized) to other organs. He was coughing, short of breath, tired, and depressed. He looked sick, with a grayish color to his skin. Doctors in Europe had told him that he had a few weeks to live and offered him chemotherapy as a last-ditch treatment. He took a plane and came to New York.

As I listened and responded to Marco I measured my every word carefully. Marco had been a heavy smoker all his life. He ate mostly red meat, pasta, wine, bread, butter, cheese, and rich deserts. He had a sweet tooth. Occasionally he ate vegetables when disguised in heavy creams.

Many cases have been reported of people who beat the odds—patients who outlive the doctor's predictions that they have days to live, sometimes by decades. "It's not over till it's over" is their war cry. But when you look at these miraculous survivors, almost all of them have one thing in common: in order to recover, they made a *radical* change from what they were doing before. Highly stressed people became serious meditators. Atheists turned into devoted followers of faith. Burger munchers transformed themselves into vegetarians.

Marco frowned when I talked about vegetable juices as a way to deliver nutrients, antioxidants, and blood alkalinizers. He thought it almost impossible to imagine whatever was left of his life without enjoying his daily wine and meat. He said he did not want to give up on life—but what he really didn't want to give up on were his habits.

This is when I said to him, "There are no incurable diseases, only incurable patients, Marco. Whatever you have been doing until now is not working for your body. So much so that it is threatening you with extinction, should you continue." This finally got his attention, and there was a sudden shift in his attitude, even in his thinking. He had an "Aha!" moment that resulted in a willingness to try something new, to consume food not as a means of pleasure but as one would consume a medication. Food as chemotherapy. Big dietary shifts offer no guarantee of curing anything. I certainly did not recommend that he turn his back on all conventional treatments. But what Marco's story exemplifies is that the most powerful tool in healing is the willingness—the open-mindedness—to try a new way when what you've been doing before is not helping you live as healthily as you could.

THE CLEAN PROGRAM

Now that you have prepared your body, your living environment, and your mind, you are ready to begin to change your life.

Clean requires a fairly radical reorientation toward food, toward eating habits, and toward the experience of hunger. The Elimination Diet will have prepared you well for this. You will be in a clearer mind to begin and will have the confidence that comes from successfully changing some old patterns.

Ready to Start: Set Your Intention

Take a few moments to ponder and set your intention. Setting your intention is the root of success. Do you "have" to do it, or do you "want" to do it? A strong desire guided by the right intention will get you started powerfully. It is very important that you set the right frame of mind and the way to think about the program you are about to start. If you think about this program as something you *have* to do for your health it will not be as powerful as thinking about it as something you *want* to do. Obligation isn't nearly as strong a driving force as desire.

We always make time for what we want. When we have a burning desire for something, we will go the extra mile or turn the planet upside down to get it. Think about it: whatever you have spent time wanting in life, you probably already have. But consider also how wanting something is usually an unconscious impulse. You see something and have to have it. The "want" is triggered almost unconsciously, and the stronger it is, the quicker you tend to get the object of your desire. Yet there are ways to cultivate or build up that desire for something—even if you feel hesitant or resistant about it at the beginning. Setting an intention is how you actively cultivate desire, so that it can propel you to success and get you over hurdles. Though these exercises seem simple, I have used them many times with patients. They can be the secret to achieving in a few short weeks a goal that may seem difficult or even impossible to you now.

Envision a different you. Close your eyes and picture your life today. How do you look and feel daily? What aspects of your well-being are you disappointed with?

What would it mean to you to look and feel younger? How might that feel?

What would it mean to your loved ones if the health issues that limit you disappeared?

How would it benefit you socially, financially, spiritually, and emotionally to live in a state of vibrant energy and mental clarity?

Visualize these possibilities; sense what they feel like. Notice how the spark of desire turns into a wildfire when you begin to feel the possibility of change. Set the intention to begin the program with commitment and to complete three weeks of it; make sure you have a strong idea of why you are doing it.

Make a Clean log. For added impact, take notes on your Clean experience. I recommend you start a Clean log to record your intentions, your current state of well-being, and your experiences and progress as you follow the Program. You will also want to take notes about the effects of foods on your system when you re-introduce them in the Completing Clean phase. This doesn't have to be a paper journal—you can make a single document on your computer to keep notes.

Note down what you visualized in the first exercise. Brief comments will be enough.

Then make a list of the results you would like to achieve by the end of the program, both physically and mentally.

This list should also include any new habits, especially around eating and drinking, that you would like to substitute for old habits that are simply not working for you anymore or are holding you back from expressing your full potential. Most people know what these are for them.

As you proceed on the program, make notes daily or every few days about how you are feeling and what is changing. Keeping a record of daily experiences is always helpful in life. But it's particularly interesting during times of accelerated transformation. Noting what is happening in your appearance, body functions, energy levels, mood, and outlook, and noting changes in any symptoms or conditions you tend to have will be useful as a point of reference in the future as you continue on the long-term journey of living health-fully. It can motivate you to embark on a future Clean program and help as you try to figure out what diet and lifestyle choices work best for you.

Take a photo of yourself. Memory is tricky—especially visual memory. Take a picture of yourself when you start the program and then at the end. You will get a kick out of seeing the transformation. Make sure both pictures are taken from the same distance and angle. Choose a simple background without too many things to distract your eyes.

Establish your support system. We are social creatures and work best when supported by others. Make sure the key people in your life know what you are up to and request their support. Enrolling a friend or partner to do Clean with you not only is fun but also will increase your chances of success.

Complete the Clean Audit in chapter 1 when you start and finish the program. A more detailed account to refresh your memory of why you were moved to do the program to begin with will help you stay on track in the future. Many of us have selective memory and filter out our bad memories. This is one of the reasons why we find ourselves dealing with the same issues over and over again. Noting what you look and feel like before you start, and then again at the end, will be your hard evidence that change happens when you commit to a program.

YOUR INSTRUCTIONS

The Clean Program requires that you do two essential things every day:

1. Eat and drink only food that is part of the Clean meals.
2. Support your body's detoxification process through simple methods and practices.

In addition, there are a few optional practices to add for maximum results. Do what your time and your natural enthusiasm allow. If you simply follow the two essentials without anything extra, you will still have excellent results.

Aim to do the full three weeks of Clean. If you do less than this, you will still benefit, and will be in a good place to go further on your next attempt.

1. FOLLOW THE CLEAN MEAL RULES

The Clean recipes were designed by Jill Pettijohn, a nurse, raw foods chef, and cleansing expert. A valued friend and trusted colleague, Jill is passionate about guiding individuals to higher levels of health and has become famous for her juice cleanses, which she delivers to her clients' doors in New York City. We have spent countless hours broadening our knowledge of cleansing and detoxification and between us we have guided many hundreds of people through detoxification programs. When I asked Jill to create a set of new recipes especially for this book, she more than met the challenge. Her forty-two recipes are not only delicious and simple for anyone to follow but also laser accurate in their supply of the key nutrients needed for detoxification.

The Strategy

Every day you will have one solid meal and two drinks or "liquid meals," a smoothie, a juice, or a soup. Plan to have the liquid meals for breakfast and dinner and the solid meal for lunch. Eating the food meal at night will be less effective, because the twelve-hour "fast" that your body will experience overnight will be most effective after a liquid dinner, as this frees up the most energy and extends the window of time for detoxification. However, if you have a business dinner or a social plan that can't get rearranged, just have the solid meal for dinner that day, with the two smoothies, juices, or soups as breakfast and lunch. The next day, return to having your solid meal at lunchtime.

Remember the twelve-hour window: the detox signal is given approximately eight hours after your last meal, and requires at least four hours to function well. If you fill up your belly late at night and eat early again the next day, you are denying the body its full detox mode. It is better to go on a little fast each night as you sleep. This is why the ritual called breakfast exists. We are literally "breaking the fast" that occurred since the previous evening. (If you do nothing more in your life than start to eat lighter in the evening and leave twelve hours between dinner one night and breakfast the next day, you will find that you have more energy and improve your overall health.) During Clean you will be required to eat liquid meals for your dinner and then not eat again until breakfast, at least twelve hours later, to let the deep cleaning happen. If dinner is at 7 p.m., breakfast should be at 7 a.m. or later; if dinner is at 11 p.m., the next meal will be at 11 a.m.

You will be making all the liquid meals yourself, choosing from the recipes in chapter 11. You have a total of twenty-one recipes to pick from: seven juices, seven smoothies, and seven blended soups. All these drinks use raw ingredients for maximum nutrition and enzyme content—even the soups, which are blended vegetable drinks that are not cooked (some can be warmed, however). If eating this way is a first for you, do not be nervous. These meals-in-a-cup are custom-designed to do the following:

- Provide the body with all the nutrients it needs.
- Deliver the nutrients in a fuel-injected way. Because they require less energy to break down, the ingredients in liquid meals can be absorbed into the bloodstream easily without much effort.
- Intelligently combine nutrients in each meal to shift your metabolism so that you feel less hungry.

To ensure that you get the right kind of nutrition in your one solid meal of the day, there are also twenty-one simple lunch recipes to choose from, some raw and some cooked: seven fish, seven meat (chicken and lamb), and seven vegetarian recipes.

You will decide which two liquid meals and which one food meal to have each day by mixing and matching the recipes as you like. The only rule is that you *always follow the basic formula of two liquid meals and one solid meal per day, with the solid meal eaten at lunchtime.*

You may snack in between as needed. Raw vegetables and some tart, fresh fruits such as blueberries and raspberries are best for this purpose because berries are low in sugar. A few raw almonds or brazil nuts are also good. You can even have an extra smoothie or juice if you feel extremely hungry (please read the section called "Dealing with Hunger"). Remember, however, that you want to avoid putting solid or liquid foods in your stomach late at night. If you want a snack after dinner, see if you can do without it and get through the night until the morning meal.

These liquid and solid meal recipes have been designed as a complete package. They will give you the full spectrum of nutrients you need for successful detoxification over the three weeks. This means that the more variety of recipes you include each week, the better. Your body will be consistently supplied with a wide array of nutrients, and you'll be sure to get the benefits of certain recipes that are engineered to supercharge you with one or two key nutrients. Variation will also make the program more fun, and it will introduce you to new ingredients and flavors that are important components of a healthy diet over the long term.

No doubt about it, though, the program will have to fit into your busy life, and it is adaptable to your needs. The following suggestions will help you tailor the program to your own lifestyle, and get the most out of Clean.

• If your time is limited, or you prefer to keep things very simple, selecting a few liquid meals and a few food meals and rotating them throughout the week will still work well.

- You do not have to always use the Clean recipes for lunch. You can create a lunch from the same simple foods you've been eating on the Elimination Diet. This might include premade items from a supermarket or a restaurant meal. Keep in mind that one of the basic principles of Clean is to avoid exposure to chemicals, so be smart about where you buy your food and buy organic for everything you can afford. Remember that all lunches should comprise basic foods without sauces, commercial dressings, or toppings. (Use the Elimination Diet list of allowed condiments and spices, as well as olive oil and lemon juice, to flavor store-bought foods.) And look at the Clean recipes to guide your portion sizes. Eating a meal for lunch that is not one of the Clean recipes should not be seen as a free pass to supersize your plate.

- The fresher the foods you eat, the more potent their nutrients. However, you won't lose out too much if you make your meals at night in order to take them to work the next day. You can also make a double portion of one liquid meal and use it for both breakfast and dinner. If you do this, keep everything in the fridge and use within two days. Juices should only be kept for one day. Note that all of the food meals can be taken with you wherever you go and eaten cold.

- As with the Elimination Diet, organic ingredients are preferable whenever possible. Even if you buy nonorganic, the combination of raw ingredients used for Clean will boost your body, especially if you are shifting from a diet that was high in cooked and or processed foods. Again, just do the best that you and your wallet can and wash everything well.

- Canned fruits and vegetables usually contain preservatives and sometimes high fructose corn syrup and salt, so avoid them at all costs. Frozen fruits are acceptable for the liquid meals, especially if they are organic.

- Your personal preferences and your environment will dictate which recipes you choose. Be adaptable. For example, the thicker, blended soups may be more appealing on cold winter mornings than the fruit smoothies, which contain ice. Remember that the thinner the liquid, the more intense the detox. Juices will promote detoxification slightly more than blended soups.

- If you don't feel a hunger for your liquid or food meal when the time for it comes, please still make and consume it, or at the very least have a half-size portion. The nutrients are necessary to keep your detoxification process supported.

• Keep the Elimination Diet "Include/Exclude List" on your fridge for the days when you are making your own lunch and refer back to it to stay on track in both eating and drinking.

Fluids

In addition to the liquid and food meals, you must drink plenty of pure water each day to enhance the detoxification work by increasing the kidney's elimination of toxins. A good estimate of how much to drink is the amount it takes to cause you to pee hourly. A typical total daily water intake is two quarts. You may add fresh lemon, cucumber, or mint to the water for flavor. During the program, avoid all caffeinated beverages. Do not drink decaffeinated coffee. Herbal teas and hot water with lemon are fine, but have them in addition to the full amount of pure water, not in place of it. Do not drink commercial fruit juices, low-calorie sodas, "natural" sodas, or energy drinks. Carbonated water adds to the acidity in the body so it is wise to exclude this also. If you're not sure what you can drink, go by the general rule that if it's not hot or cold water, and if it's in a bottle with a name on it, it's probably to be avoided. It's only for a few days of your life, so for now, keep it simple and pure.

Day 1

Breakfast: Green Smoothie. Hot water and lemon, or herbal tea
Mid-morning: Snack or herbal tea (optional)
Lunch: Steamed Bass with Fennel, Parsley, and Capers
Mid-afternoon: Snack or herbal tea (optional)
Dinner: Chilled Cucumber Soup with Mint
Drink plenty of pure water all day.

Day 2

Breakfast: Carrot, Beet, Cabbage, and Watercress Juice; hot water with lemon, or herbal tea
Mid-morning: Snack or herbal tea (optional)
Lunch: Stir-Fry Vegetables with Buckwheat Noodles
Mid-afternoon: Snack or herbal tea (optional)
Dinner: Fennel and Apple Juice
Drink plenty of pure water all day.

Day 3

Breakfast: Energy Smoothie with Almond Butter and Cardamom
Mid-morning: Snack or herbal tea (optional)
Lunch: Plain roast chicken and salad from supermarket
Mid-afternoon: Snack or herbal tea (optional)
Dinner: Energy Smoothie with Almond Butter and Cardamom
Drink plenty of pure water all day.

Day 4

Breakfast: Easy Pineapple and Avocado Gazpacho
Mid-morning: Snack or herbal tea (optional)
Lunch: A piece of steamed salmon and steamed mixed vegetables made at home
Mid-afternoon: Snack or herbal tea (optional).
Dinner: Green Juice
Drink plenty of pure water all day.

When all this is put into practice, each person's intake of Clean meals is unique to him or her. It may look very different week to week, or you may find a formula with the amount of variety you can handle, and stick to it for the three weeks. A few days of Clean will typically look something like the chart above.

A weekly planning and preparation chart is provided on p. 192 to help you organize what you plan to make and what you need to buy.

Your Clean Detox Nutrients

Nature provides all the nutrients you need for full-functioning detox. It's up to you, however, to select them and get them into your body. The Clean recipes include all the nutrients you'll need over the next few weeks as you switch detox onto "high." Your snacks and any "off the menu" lunches can also be selected with these nutritional needs in mind. Use the "Detoxification Nutrients" chart (see appendix) during the program and afterward, to ensure that you fund all the needs of your busy liver by including many of these foods every week.

Clean delivers its maximum benefits when a few easy-to-find natural *supplements* are added into your daily intake. Though they're not obligatory, I highly recommend them, and they are not expensive. Buy

The Clean Kit includes:

- Shake powders made from brown rice protein that contain all the nutrients, vitamins, minerals, antioxidants, and phytonutrients needed to support daily cell metabolism and the additional work of detoxification, specifically phase 1 and phase 2 of liver detoxification.
- A high concentration of probiotics to reinoculate your intestinal tract with a healthy, viable flora.
- A combination of herbal antimicrobials that will eliminate yeast and pathogenic bacteria in most cases, and an herbal supplement that will regulate insulin peaks and lows, thus eliminating cravings as well as facilitating fat burning.

The cost of this kit is an investment, but it is reasonable and it is a convenient option for those who otherwise would not do the Clean program. (See appendix "Clean Resources" for more information on how to order the Clean Kit.)

the best brands you can find, asking your local health food store for guidance. (Online vitamin stores often have low prices.) All of these nutrients are available as part of the Clean Kit. Visit www.cleanprogram .com. Good supplements should be thought of as health insurance. For a little extra investment upfront they save money over the long term on doctor's visits, prescription drugs, and missed workdays. They'll add years to your life, especially when used as part of a detoxification program like Clean—and they'll add life to your years.

Fiber plays an important role in elimination support (see the next section, "Enhancing Elimination") because it absorbs water and creates bulk, which triggers the peristaltic movement of your intestines and promotes bowel elimination. Fiber sequesters (pulls out) toxic waste that the intestines keep clearing from the blood, making sure that the toxins don't get reabsorbed. Fiber feeds the good bacteria, promoting a healthy environment in the intestines. It also captures cholesterol and prevents its excess absorption, while giving you a feeling of fullness, thereby limiting overeating. For all these reasons and more, high-fiber diets are associated with a decreased incidence of colon cancer and heart disease. Though the Clean program is filled with fruits and vegetables, it may contain less roughage than you are used to. Most people benefit from adding some form of fiber to the program. Look for natural fiber products containing ingredients like psyllium husks and psyllium seed, prune fiber, guar gum, and flax seeds. Bentonite clay is used in cleansing-detox programs to further bind to toxic chemicals including heavy metals and to reduce gas in the intestines. Fiber should be adjusted to the number and consistency of bowel movements. Most quality products come with dosing instructions.

Probiotics are a very valuable tool in the restoration of the hundreds of different species of good intestinal bacteria. There are lots of good probiotics supplements for sale, some of which need to be refrigerated once opened; make sure yours has at least 15 billion organisms per dose. Read the instructions carefully. One dose a day should be enough during Clean, but there is no downside that I know of to taking more.

Antimicrobials help kill the pathogenic (bad) bacteria. Many of the foods in the Clean recipes such as garlic, lemon, olive oil, onions, broccoli, coconut oil, and many of the spices have antimicrobial properties. But sometimes the intestinal flora is in such state of disarray (dysbiosis) that it needs a little heavier artillery to clean the territory so that the good bacteria can take up residence once more. A smart measure is to take one or more of the following during Clean. *Concentrated oil of oregano* is especially potent against yeast (look for it as a pill or essential oil). A *clove of garlic* can be eaten daily, raw. (Slice it and place it between thin apple slices if you prefer). This will not only help to eliminate bad bacteria, yeast, and parasites; it will also help regulate blood sugar levels, enhance fat burning, reduce hunger sensations, lower cholesterol, relieve arthritic pain, and reduce bowel gas. If this is unappealing, *garlic pills* are an inexpensive and easy way to ingest effective amounts of garlic. You may find an herbal antimicrobial that combines several different antimicrobial herbs and roots. Berberine, licorice root, rhubarb root, skullcap root, coptis root, ginger root, sage leaf, and thyme oil are some of the ingredients I look for.

Olive oil taken at night will lubricate your intestines, improve bowel elimination, provide anti-inflammatory fats, kill germs and enhance fat burning, stimulate the gallbladder and liver to move bile clearing the liver system, promote bone formation, inhibit blood clot formation, and promote hormonal balance. Take two tablespoons before bed every night and follow with water and lemon.

Finally, try to include a *liver support* product during your Clean program. These can be a single ingredient or a combination of ingredients. The most common available liver support herbs are milk thistle (sylimarin), N acetyl cysteine, dandelion root, and wormwood leaf. Ask the staff at your health food store for advice; many salespeople seem to have Ph.D.-level knowledge of liver support preparations!

FAQs About Doing the Clean Program

Q: I work out and train hard physically. Can I still do Clean?

A: Yes. Recreational and competitive athletes alike have successfully done Clean, losing weight while upping their performance. It is not recommended to do Clean during intensive precompetition training, but at any other time you can keep training while on the program. Double or even triple the servings of your liquid meals. Use more of the soups and energy smoothies than juices and make sure your lunchtime meal includes lean protein, healthy fat such as avocado or coconut, and some of the allowed grains from the Elimination Diet.

Q: I drop weight easily and am already slightly underweight. What should I do?

A: You can safely do the program. Weight loss is always greater amongst those who need to lose weight as the body is looking to find its best state of balance. Any pounds you do lose, you can put on strategically when you are done by eating plenty of good fats, clean proteins, and whole grains. However, it will help you to double up on your liquid meals during Clean, and to make sure your daily meals are satisfying in portion size. Include nuts in your snacks.

Q: I am too busy to prepare the Clean drinks and smoothies. Can I still do Clean?

A: *When patients' schedules are so busy that they have no time to make their own liquid meals, I suggest an alternative option. The Clean Kit (www.cleanprogram.com) contains powdered shake mixes and a supply of supplements that delivers all the enzymes, herbs, and nutrients needed to successfully complete the work of cleansing and repair, while you eat the daily food meal from the Clean recipes or the general Elimination Diet. After testing many products over the years, I now rely on a combination of products from a reliable manufacturer that has proved to be highly effective and totally safe. All the products are made from natural ingredients and are free of added chemicals.*

2. SUPPORT YOUR BODY'S DETOXIFICATION

The second essential instruction for doing the Clean program is to support your body's detoxification process. There are many ways to do this.

Enhancing Elimination

The Clean program depends on effective elimination for much of its success. With less energy dedicated to digesting, absorbing, transporting and assimilating foods, the body will be redirecting its energy toward "catching up" with inner cleaning. As it shifts into releasing toxins from cells and tissues, your job is to support the channels of elimination so that these waste products can now make their way out. It is simple to do, and it is very important. Without this step, you won't see all the benefits—and in some cases, if you ignore elimination, you can create discomfort and even health problems. The channels of elimination include the skin, the lungs, the kidneys, the bowels, and the circulatory system, which connects them all through two subsystems, the blood vessels and the lymphatic system. Here are tools to enhance their function. Use them individually or in combination until you are successful.

BOWEL ELIMINATION

Many of the toxins and most of the mucus that is pulled out of the tissues and captured from the blood get eliminated through the bowels, bound up in feces. Facilitating the movement of this waste material through the intestines is crucial at all times, but especially during a detox program, when it is very common to see this mucus mixed in with, or surrounding, your stools. It is sticky, so naturally, can cause constipation; you must do whatever you can to support daily, generous, bowel movements. Fiber supplements, which help grab the toxins and move everything toward the exit, might not always be sufficient to keep things moving as quickly and as efficiently as you need during this deep-clean program.

This toxic mix has a tendency to stick to the intestinal wall in a layer of plaque that thickens as the hours go by. When it's not released in healthy feces, this constipated mix lets toxins get reabsorbed and then digested by the pathogenic bacteria in the intestinal walls. They in turn will emit their even stronger toxins and exacerbate the condition of dysbiosis. Avoid constipation even for one day during Clean. Use your fiber supplements, drink lots of pure water, and take gentle to moderate exercise to promote daily, generous bowel movements. If they don't happen easily, take herbal laxatives every night. Dr. Schulze's Intestinal Formula #1 is the most potent one available, almost guaranteed to make you eliminate consistently thanks to its mix of wild harvested herbs, including senna and cascara sagrada (available from www.herbdoc.com). Swiss Kriss is another effective and trusted brand, readily available at health food stores. In both cases, read the instructions and take as many doses as necessary to achieve the goal of consistent elimination. Even if they give you mild diarrhea occasionally, do not be concerned unless it is constant and it dehydrates you. In this case, cut back on the amount of laxatives you take or leave them out for a day to restore balance.

There is no set number of bowel movements a day that everyone must have, whether in daily life or during a detox program. "Optimal elimination" means as much as is necessary to dispose of the materials that will affect the system negatively. With a good, healthy diet, free of toxins, one should eliminate feces after every meal. Most of us eliminate much less often than that— in general we are a constipated population—and it's now considered normal to have one movement a day, with many people having less than that. In its healthiest states, the stool should have the color and consistency of peanut butter (though some healthy foods like dark green vegetables turn it darker). When your stool is more solid than this consistency, it is an early sign of constipation. A healthy stool shouldn't smell in a way that urges the evacuation of the bathroom and it shouldn't take too much effort to eliminate.

If a day goes by without a bowel movement, try taking a dose of castor oil, the oldest trick in the world for encouraging the release of toxicity and mucus. It works as well today as it did a hundred years ago, when family doctors used it as a remedy for practically every situation. Start with half a shot glass of it followed by a glass of water with lemon juice. Wait thirty to forty-five minutes to see if this promotes a bowel movement. If it does not work, repeat. If necessary, repeat again until the bowels begin to move. The release can be intense at times, so you will want to avoid doing this while busy at work or far away from a bathroom.

Colonic hydrotherapy. To effectively boost the removal of the mucoid plaque that gets pulled out during Clean, use colonic hydrotherapy during the program. Contrary to what many Western-trained physicians may say, colonics are very safe and beneficial when done with the right therapist. During the treatment, pure water is delivered at low pressure into the colon and then drawn out, which irrigates the colon and helps it release waste matter. There are two kinds, the open system and closed system, both of which are hygienic, discreet, and not uncomfortable. You can research which one you like better. A detoxification program is the time when colonics are most beneficial, especially to those with a history of constipation. You can have as many treatments during Clean as you like, depending on your budget and schedule. (I've even had patients who got them daily during their detox.)

Enemas are a self-administered way of irrigating the lower colon; they are helpful too, and may be used during Clean, though they do not work as deeply as colonics.

When you switch from a poor diet to a better one, better bowel movements are of the earliest benefits you will get. It can be a major part of the relief and improvement that comes from a detoxification program, both physically and mentally. And there is no reason for this benefit to be lost after you finish Clean, provided that you continue to eat and drink foods that do not cause irritation and mucus production in your system, keep the intestinal flora in good repair, and maintain the twelve-hour window at night.

OTHER TYPES OF ELIMINATION

The bowels are by no means the only avenue of elimination that your body uses. All types of elimination need to be supported during Clean, and afterward.

Kidney Elimination. Make sure you urinate frequently during Clean. After the liver does its hard work of transforming fat-loving toxic molecules into water-soluble ones, they need to be filtered out of the body by the kidneys and eliminated via your urine. Drink enough water that you pee every hour. If urination happens less than that, you are not drinking enough water. Lemon, cucumbers, coconut, and other ingredients used in the Clean recipes are natural diuretics that will help this process too.

Lung Elimination. Breathing is a crucial method for releasing toxins. When you exhale carbon dioxide, you are getting rid of acidity in the blood. (Remember the carbonic acid made by the little factories of your cells? This becomes carbon dioxide gas.) Make a point of using your lungs fully and deeply; visualize how each inhale is supplying you with the number one most essential nutrient you need to live, oxygen, and each exhale is an essential way of offloading the waste material that must be removed. Automatically, your breaths will become fuller and calmer.

Many people do breathing exercises to eliminate toxins from both the nervous system and the thinking brain. A simple exercise involves putting attention on the breath in a mindful way for a few minutes. Start by breathing in and out through the nose, letting the belly inflate and then the back and chest expand on the inhale; then letting the chest and back contract but keeping the chest lifted, and then letting the belly flatten on the exhale. Keep the rhythm as regular and as slow as you can. Most important, keep your attention focused on your breath. Be aware at all times if you are inhaling or exhaling. Notice how the moment you take your attention away from breathing, the autopilot kicks in—you will continue to breathe, but your attention will be elsewhere, most likely in thoughts, and soon your breaths get short and shallow. Each time you notice this, gently bring your attention back to your breath. This exercise can be done anywhere, at any time, even in the middle of an important meeting. It will be cleaning out the lungs while quieting and clearing the mind.

Skin Elimination. Sweating is another mechanism for eliminating toxins. In a healthy person, the skin is usually spared the job of eliminating heavy-duty toxins and mucus, and mainly releases excess water, minerals, and salts. But if your bowels are not doing their job, the body will recruit the other organs of elimination to compensate. If this happens, your skin pays the price with breakouts and problems that cosmetics and creams applied to the surface don't fix. During a detox program, the skin might have to do some extra work at the beginning. Skin rashes or breakouts during the first few days of Clean are not uncommon; they are a sign that accelerated detoxification is happening. (Of course, use your common sense. Nobody knows your body better than you, so if at any point any of the effects of the

program seem alarmingly abnormal, consult your doctor or preferably a health-care practitioner who is familiar with the detoxification process.)

Taking saunas maximizes elimination via the skin
during Clean, especially infrared saunas, a powerful
method for boosting sweating. Steam rooms can be
helpful as well, although they are less effective than
saunas. Skin brushing is another simple, cheap, and
effective practice that will help elimination and can
easily be done daily during Clean. Your skin is constantly scaling off dead cells, but you'll want to speed
the process during a detox to prevent the dead skin
from blocking your pores. Finally, hot-cold plunges
are a detoxification secret weapon.

The most effective sauna is an infrared sauna. This
newer technology heats up the user's body instead of
heating the air with steam like a traditional Finnish
sauna. It creates radiant heat from long light waves
that are not visible by the eye (like sunlight diffused
by clouds). These rays penetrate more deeply below
the skin than the heat of a regular sauna, exciting the
fat molecules into vibration so that they release toxins. It also boosts circulation, which is desirable at all
times, but especially during Clean, as the blood needs
to carry toxins efficiently to the liver for processing.
Those used to regular saunas will probably find that

they sweat more in the infrared version. However, regular saunas will do if you can't find infrared. In both cases, remember to rehydrate during and after the sauna with lots of pure water.

Skin brushing involves using a soft, natural-bristle brush with a long handle on your dry skin, before a bath or shower. These brushes can be found in health food stores and some drugstores. Use long strokes and circular strokes to gently "scrub" the dry skin, from feet to head, including the front and back of the body, the arms, and neck, always moving inward toward the heart. Do this for several minutes daily if possible. Go gently on thinner-skinned areas and use more pressure in thicker-skinned areas such as your back and the soles of the feet. A loofah works too. In addition to removing dead skin cells, you are stimulating the all-important lymph system, the hormonal system, and glands. For best results follow this with a hot-cold plunge or shower. If you need to moisturize the skin afterward, try using a small amount of natural oil like sesame or coconut oil instead of a chemical-filled drugstore product.

In a *hot-cold plunge,* you alternate between hot and cold water repeatedly to boost circulation and detoxification. Your skin is your largest organ: it contains miles of arterioles and venules that are filled with blood. These vessels relax and dilate with heat and contract with cold. When this relax/contract pattern happens, your skin pumps almost as much blood as your heart. You don't need to go to a spa or bathhouse to do it. In your shower, turn the water as hot as you can tolerate for one minute and then as cold as you can go for one minute and repeat this 4 or 5 times. Doing this daily is an easy way to support the skin's detoxification function.

EXERCISE

Exercise boosts the effectiveness of all the elimination channels at once. It increases circulation of both blood and lymph. It makes you sweat. It stimulates the bowels to eliminate. It makes you breathe more heavily and deeply. It relaxes your mind and puts you in the present. It burns calories, and, last but not least, it releases endorphins, the feel-good hormones that are nature's antidote to stress and worry. Use your common sense. Don't run a marathon during detoxification, especially during the first few days of your first Clean. Until you get familiar with what your body is doing and how it feels, take exercise slowly and increase the intensity gradually; start by walking more and taking the stairs. Longer periods of exercise will speed up your metabolism and help with weight loss. Scientific data show concretely how exercise helps reverse most chronic diseases. Make sure you include some form of exercise daily, during Clean and beyond.

Yoga. Some forms of exercise have extra detoxification power. Hatha yoga's series of twists and bends massage the organs and promote their good functioning. Jumping exercises like jump rope and mini-trampoline (also called rebounding) are favorites on detox programs because they stimulate blood and lymphatic circulation.

In addition to being relaxing and nurturing, *massage* helps release toxins by boosting the circulation of lymph, the fluid that carries waste, debris, toxins, and sick cells through the lymph nodes. These "healing stations" act like filters, processing and removing sick cells and fighting viruses and bacteria. Deep-tissue massage works best for detoxification purposes, but any massage technique will help during Clean.

As long as you support the essentials of elimination—bowel, kidney, and basic exercise—you'll get Clean no matter how much or little of these support practices you do. There are varying degrees of Clean—it's sort of comparable to taking a shower without soap, with soap, or with a salt-scrub, soap, and loofah. Do what feels right to you on your first program, trying a few new measures whenever you can.

Rest and Sleep

One of our biggest health challenges is the lack of enough time for resting and repairing. Americans tend to be sleep-deprived; let Clean be an opportunity to change this. Energy levels always fluctuate during a detoxification program. Your body may crave sleep at the beginning, making you more tired earlier than usual. Allow yourself to get as much rest as you need and go to bed early because sleep is when much of the important repair work is done. A natural correction of fatigue tends to occur during the program, at which point it is normal to find yourself waking up earlier than usual, without the normal tiredness or desire to stay in bed. Make adequate rest as much of a priority as you can, even if it means cutting out some TV, reading, or socializing.

QUANTUM DETOXIFICATION: CLEANING THE MIND

East, West, Stress: Older traditions of health care are based on the idea that when conditions in the mind shift, so do conditions in the body. Harmony in the body is greatly dependent on balance in the mind. In India the single word *amma* denotes all toxins, whether physical or mental, that accumulate and throw off health. Most Eastern medicine practitioners know that by helping the patient establish a cleanliness or purity of awareness, orderliness of body is created as a mirror reflection of that order.

The Western medical point of view acknowledges the connection between mind and body more than it realizes. Scientists can observe and measure how continued stress responses literally change the biochemistry of the body (the fight-or-flight stress response floods you with cortisol) and also change behavior (such as pushing you into unhealthy eating and sleeping habits). Any doctor who works shifts in the emergency room can tell you that Monday mornings are characterized by a wave of heart attack and stroke patients, marking exactly the time when weekend fun and rest shifts to work-related stress and worry. From an integrative or open-minded medicine point of view, we can combine the two understandings and say that stress, anger, or disappointment experienced at the level of thought and feeling are so potentially corrosive that they sometimes have to *make themselves visible* as physical symptoms in order to get your attention. These stressful thoughts find a pathway to the weakest part of your body and begin to disrupt functioning.

For all these reasons, detoxification does not limit itself to the aspects of toxicity we can see, touch, or measure. It also means getting rid of bad thoughts and

feelings and letting go of negative relationships, emotions, jobs, or even toxic governments. It means much
more than just cleaning your body and maximizing
the liver function. It includes meditation and clearing
and calming your mind. What we find is that detoxification at the physical level facilitates detoxification in
its quantum counterpart, and vice versa.

Clean presents an opportunity to change some patterns
for a few weeks. This includes changing the patterns of
the mind. If some of the biggest obstacles to radiant well-
being are the quantum toxins of stress and endless thinking, then one of the most important acts any of us can do
to achieve better health is to engage in *quantum detoxification:* clearing the debris and toxic waste that fills up the
mind on a daily basis, and recapturing some of that lost
attention that drains out of our brains in random, repeti-
tive thinking. You can start this easily and simply with a
few practices that I ask my patients to include in their
three-week program.

Today's new age ideas have got everyone striving
for positive thinking. "Think positive" is a universal goal. But though positive thinking is much more
pleasant than negative thinking, it also consumes our
attention, our life energy, and can be the leak that
causes disease or prevents healing. Becoming present, reclaiming our attention from the thinking mind,

whether it is thinking positive or negative thoughts, is what will ultimately allow this energy to be redirected into something other than generating thoughts.

ATTENTION, THE ENERGY OF LIFE

Understanding the true meaning of "attention" is the key to quantum detoxification. Right now, as you continue to read this page, put some of your attention on your right hand. Don't stop reading. Do it at the same time. Feel your right hand. You don't need to look at it; you can feel it while you read. Feel the temperature in your hand; feel any dampness there, feel the edges of the fingers touching each other. Now think of this: Your hand was there before I asked you to put your attention on it, yet you weren't feeling it. You weren't aware of it. Your hand became part of your awareness the instant you put your attention on it. Your hand becomes your felt reality at that time, it becomes your experience. So we can conclude that wherever your attention is at any given moment will determine your experience at that moment.

The total experience of your life is the sum total of every one of those moments.

Now consider this. In order to put that attention into your hand, you activated a cable made of neurons cells) that connects your brain to your hand. The charge you are sending down and up this cable, that just a moment before was idle and unused, is literally a charge of electricity. It is a current of electrons, which in turn, as quantum physics revealed, is just energy, or light. This energy was being used for something else right before you used it to send it down that cable. Everything is in constant flow. The instant you decide to use this energy to connect your brain with your hand, you are actually redistributing or reallocating energy (just like with the digestion-detox systems). You are claiming this attention from wherever it was going before and are now choosing to direct it down the neuron cable to your hand. More than likely, this attention was flowing upward into the thinking mind, splashing out like water from an overfilled pool. Instead of connecting your brain with your hand, it was connecting the brain with thoughts and it was doing so automatically, by default. When you are shifting your attention by choice, you are using your will.

When attention is flowing into thoughts, you become not present to the reality before you in each moment. Thoughts are in the past or the future; they are in imaginary places and situations. Stuck in their grip, you become "lost in thought." Curiously, your body does not know. It continues to react as if your thoughts were real. Get wrapped up in thoughts about a fight you had with someone, and adrenaline will be released to prepare you for fight or flight. Your body is actually making your quantum thoughts a physical reality, and paying the price.

When your attention is flowing into your hand, it stays in the present. Your hand is right here in the now. It's not the thought of a hand, past or future. This is the same for any part of your body; it exists in the present. Keeping your attention on your hand or any body part is a way of anchoring yourself in the present. Those cables you are using are now actively transporting electrons. Since you reclaimed these electrons back from the thinking mind, your thoughts naturally diminish in number and intensity and you start silencing your mind. Meanwhile there is friction in the new cables that are being used. Heat is generated; the cables warm up; the frequency of vibration increases. Your electrons are, ultimately, impulses of light; by sending them into your body, you are literally enlightening yourself.

Reclaiming the constant flow of attention that is flowing into thoughts and sending it through other pathways is the art and practice of becoming present. It is a powerful tool for quantum detoxification, one that starts with the individual but ultimately, one person at a time, redresses the collective insanity of toxic emotions, toxic relationships, and toxic lifestyles that know no borders. Living this way requires you to retrain new mental pathways. It requires conscious effort and is very hard at the beginning. But with time and constant practice it becomes easier and easier, until a new habit is formed, that of always being present. This practice is one form of meditation.

Here are some practical tools for thinking about quantum toxicity and practices to do during your Clean program.

Five-Minute Meditation. There are many schools of meditation worldwide that offer hundreds of different meditation techniques. The following technique is one that has helped me enormously, and I recommend it to my patients. You only need five minutes. It sounds like very little, but it takes great will and effort to sit quietly for even that long. The best time to do it is as soon as you wake up in the morning, before the thinking locomotive of your brain starts up at full speed. But doing it at any time of the day or evening is better than not doing it at all.

This meditation exercise is very powerful when done consistently. After doing five minutes every day, you may start noticing a shift in your awareness. Maybe you have a brief pause before your old automatic responses

Five-Minute Meditation

Sit up in a chair with your back straight. Place your feet under your knees. Rest the palms of your hands on your thighs and relax your arms. Look straight ahead but try not to focus anywhere in particular. Instead, notice everything in the room at once. Take a deep breath and start feeling your feet. Feel them touching the floor or the inside of your shoes. Feel the temperature, the humidity; feel the texture of your socks. Feel your feet intensely from inside. Do not "think" about them, just feel them, sense them.

After a few breaths, move your attention to your calves and legs. Feel and sense these in the same way for several breaths. Then move your attention from body part to body part, first to your thighs, then your bottom against the chair, then to your abdomen and lower back, your chest and upper back, your shoulders, your arms, your hands, your neck, face, and lastly your head. Then let your awareness cover your whole body at the same time. The idea is to "scan" your body with your attention, stopping for a few breaths on each part. This practice will strengthen your ability to intentionally direct your attention and hold it in place.

You may notice that the moment you sit down, you start remembering things and feel the urge to

➤

act on them. This is part of the process. When those thoughts come and try to steal your attention away from your body, simply say silently to yourself, "Thank you for sharing" and direct your attention back to your body. If you feel discomfort or frustration and want to stop, just keep sitting calmly. Know that the discomfort you feel is not caused by the exercise itself. It's what happens when you become aware of your baseline state, that underlying anxiety of which you are typically not aware when the outside world is at full volume and your attention is far from your body. Becoming aware of this underlying state is the first step toward dissolving it, and claiming back the energy it consumes.

When you find yourself consumed in thinking, if for a second you can separate your attention from your thoughts, ask yourself, "Who is deciding that these thoughts appear? If I had a choice, would I be thinking them?" If your answer is no, and you understand that these thoughts just "popped" into your mind, grabbing and consuming your attention to the point of taking you away from where you are and whom you are with, say to your thoughts, "Thank you for sharing!" and immediately direct your attention to go somewhere in the present. For example, you can put your attention on your feet this time. Again, this does not mean "think" about your feet, but "feel" them. This small "shock" of awareness erodes the habitual pathways of attention that lead away from the present and into distracted thoughts. Do it randomly and as often as you can.

This technique can also be used in the middle of any stressful situation in which you are not alone, like a business meeting or a job interview. Nervousness comes from the unconscious thinking process of interpreting, judging, measuring, and expecting. This process takes attention. By directing your attention into your body or breath, you reclaim this unwanted use of attention and eliminate the effects it causes. It may be hard to remember to do this in difficult situations. Start with easy ones. Then try to do it in harder and harder ones. My personal experience is that if I have the presence of mind for a split second to remember and start doing it, immediately the energy of the situation shifts, usually for the better. When you become more present, the others in the room feel it as well. They may not be aware of exactly why, but they feel a sense of relief. More trust and more respect is the consequence. And the business meeting has a better chance of going well.

kick in, including reactions that tend to get you in trouble or cause more stress around you. It's an opportunity to not contribute to more toxic thinking and relating. You become more present, and people around you may start noticing it as well. Time seems to be slower; you may find you can do more in the same amount of time than before.

If you can't instantly switch off your mind and feel the bliss that the yogis and Zen monks talk about, do not conclude that meditation is not for you. As my own teachers told me, this may not come for years, or even lifetimes of practice. But doing this exercise for five minutes every morning, for twenty-one days, will give you a taste of the transformation that is possible if you follow a consistent meditation practice. What this looks and feels like is different for everyone; it's as hard to explain as the taste of a strawberry. You simply have to taste it yourself.

Meditation in Action. Many studies have shown that regular meditation practices greatly improve physical health. There are quantifiable reasons for this; there is a reduction in stress-related body chemistry and happier hormones get released, the body gets a chance to deeply rest and heal. But you can also think of it this way. You are reclaiming some attention or energy that is getting wasted or lost—in this case, thoughts that are streaming

The Art of Conscious Thinking

Along my journey I have met some remarkable people. One in particular was key in helping me "order my library." On my return from India, I was somewhat confused. I had dived into the practice of meditation and flirted with hatha yoga. I had read the teachings of many spiritual teachers and could almost see the common thread that tied them all together. But as soon as I tried to talk about it, I clearly realized I didn't quite "get" it.

I met Hugo Cory by chance one day at Café Café, a trendy coffee shop in Soho's Greene Street. Sitting with him and discussing these ideas for half an hour was one of the most enlightening experiences of my life. I discovered that he meets with clients in an office on Madison Avenue and 67th Street and I began to work with him. Hugo describes his work as developing integrity and character through the learning and practicing of Self-Mastery. In this work, the simplest advice, which sounds almost superficial during casual conversation, is a powerful tool for transformation. "Stop complaining," he says, and then remains silent looking right into your eyes. As if downloading a program over a high-speed Internet

➤

connection, I saw with a jolt how any complaint is really the expression of a negative emotion or state. It gives the complainer a sense of immediate relief, even pleasure. This is perhaps the reason why it is such a common practice worldwide.

I realized that 90 percent of the time, people complain about everything and everyone. The weather, the government, the economy, their jobs, the basketball game, their spouse, the cost of gas. Complaints are not always obvious. There are masters of disguise who make them sound like a joke, or make them so intellectually complex that they fool almost everyone. Except Hugo. His radar for the subtle energy of complaining has become so refined that it surprises people who truly believe they never complain (when he points it out to them without judgment). He explains that negative emotions create a certain inner turmoil that generates a type of pressure. Complaining is like an exhaust pipe in a car, it lets out the pressure, relieving the complainer in the short term. But this negative energy pollutes your environment and is doubly toxic to the people who are listening. The almost victim-like quality that this energy carries generates a curious phenomenon. Most complainers expect you to join them in their complaint. Even if it is with a nod of your head, or a lowering of your eyelids. Most people are so blind to this toxicity that they are eager to join the complainer, sometimes going as far as to engage in criticism of someone they barely know. The apparent camaraderie that is generated by this interaction gives the one who joins the complainer a sense of immediate pleasure as well.

Hugo pointed out, and I confirmed by my own observation, that almost without exception, complainers and those who join them later on, when alone, feel depleted, somewhat depressed. Most never put these two dots together and have no way of ever breaking this cycle of quantum toxicity, both personal and environmental. Over the years, I have witnessed several people completely transform their lives and end eternal cycles of drama while working with Hugo on this one aim alone, to stop and master all complaints and expression of negative emotions. Along the way, some of them saw the resolution of apparently completely unrelated health issues that were resistant to conventional and alternative treatment approaches. Take this idea and run with it. First observe and see if you notice yourself complaining. Then attempt to stop complaining about anything. Learn about Hugo's work by visiting his Web site at www.hugocory.com.

out of your mind with no real purpose or direction—and redirecting it to your body, where attention is often needed most. The sages say, "What we put our attention on, grows." Let that object be your vitality and health.

DEALING WITH HUNGER

Dealing with hunger is a part of Quantum Detoxification. An obvious issue that comes up when food intake is reduced is, of course, hunger. The anxiety people feel concerning hunger can scare them away from even starting a detoxification program. The real battle is usually with the mind and emotions. The body can go for days without food if needed; it adjusts itself quite easily to changes in intake. It benefits so hugely from the break in digestion that if the body were completely in charge of things, there wouldn't be a problem. But the mind can be very resistant, until, several days into Clean, it learns that you can function well and feel good on two liquid meals or juices and one solid meal a day.

When hunger hits you during the Clean program, it's not an obstacle. It's actually an excellent opportunity. Redefining what hunger means to you is one of the most important and life-changing aspects of Clean. Examining, questioning, and redefining that thing we call hunger will free you from the traps you might be in around food. Maybe you eat too much of it and are overweight, like the majority of the population today. Maybe you eat the wrong kinds of it, and your moods and physical functioning suffer, but you lack the discipline to change your diet. Or you eat without awareness, because food fills some other roles in your life beyond nourishment. Almost everyone in some way uses food to provide more than just "building blocks" for the body and brain. This is a chance to contemplate what purpose food really serves in your life.

As hunger creeps up during the day or evening, ask yourself, what does being hungry actually mean? Do you really know? Have you ever *truly* been hungry, or have you ever actually been "starving"—the word we unconsciously use when we're telling our friends that we really feel like eating *right this minute*? Probably the truth is that you have not.

That body sensation that you recognize as "being hungry" and that makes you eat whenever you feel it coming on may have nothing to do with your body's actual need for calories. Most likely, if you just stay with it and watch it, it will disappear within minutes. How many times has the following scenario happened to you? You're driving and you suddenly feel hungry. You're starving, in fact, and you are certain that you

Digestion Starts in the Mouth

Tip: Chew all your food well, even your liquid meals. Chewing triggers the production and release of saliva, which then mixes with the food, initiating its digestion, preparing the alkalinity of the stomach, killing germs, and lubricating the swallowed food for a smoother transit through the esophagus. It also releases brain chemicals that decrease the feeling of hunger (which is why dieters enjoy chewing gum).

need to eat immediately. But there's nowhere to stop on the highway. So you keep driving. Twenty minutes later, when you finally approach a rest stop, you realize you've forgotten about that hunger. The intensity of the thought had faded and your body was quite able to continue functioning. Knowing that this happens naturally can help you during your program. When the sensation of hunger rises up in you, if it is mild or moderate, drink a glass of water slowly. This can often dispel the urgent need for food until your thoughts change. If the sensation is so strong as to unsettle you, try this exercise.

Take a moment before reacting to the hunger to ask yourself, what is it that I'm feeling right now? This thing

I'm calling hunger, where is it? Is it in my stomach, my guts, my chest, my heart—where is that body sensation? Then ask, what is the sensation? Everyone has a different description of this experience that they name "hungry." Stay with it, watch it, and try to distinguish its qualities. Is it hot or cold, does it feel like pain or pressure, is it fixed or moving, is it in waves or is it constant? By asking yourself those questions, you are directing your attention to this body sensation; it's literally putting the light to it so you can see it better. You'll probably notice that the sensation is not actually the body crying out for nutrients. It might actually be a very different kind of need that has nothing to do with food: a need for company, for contact, for forgiveness, for acknowledgement, for purpose, or for security. Once this is noticed, you can decide to take no action around filling the belly, and just wait until your next Clean meal or snack. You can also decide whether you need to take action on that underlying need or not (for example by calling a friend or doing something comforting for yourself). Sometimes a simple walk can be enough to change the environment; what you were "hungry" for was stimulation or a change, and that didn't have to come from food or drink.

When we begin to bring this kind of attention to hunger, it often reveals how we habitually "kill" hunger at first sight. Sometimes it's because we are so

The Clean Program At-a-Glance

Copy this chart and put it somewhere where you will see it daily. You can also download it from www.cleanprogram.com.

The Essentials: Do These Daily

1. Plan and prepare your three meals: Liquid meal for breakfast; solid food meal for lunch; liquid meal for dinner, with any supplements you've selected.

2. Follow the Elimination Diet guidelines for everything you consume.

3. Leave a twelve-hour window between the last meal of one day and the first meal of the next. Try not to snack in between.

4. Make sure you have a bowel movement before the end of the day. If this doesn't happen spontaneously, make it happen with laxatives or castor oil.

5. Drink enough pure water to cause you to pee often. If more than one hour has gone by without peeing, you are not drinking enough.

6. Move. Walk. Take the stairs. Jump. Incorporate more movement into your day, as often and for as long as you possibly can. Park your car two blocks away from your destination. Get off the subway or the bus a stop before you should and walk the rest of the way.

7. Rest. Get enough sleep. And breathe deeply all day long.

The Optional Activities

Do as many of the following activities as you can during each week of Clean:

1. Exercise. In addition to your increased daily motion, more deliberate exercise practices will pay off big time. Start slowly and increase gradually as the days go by.

2. Five-minute meditation exercise. Clean your mind and emotions as you clean your body.

3. Colonics. Daily bowel movements will do the work. Colonics will accelerate the process.

4. Skin brushing. Spend a few minutes removing dead skin cells before your shower.

5. Hot-cold treatments. In the shower, use alternating hot and cold water to power up circulation and detoxification.

6. Infrared sauna. Sweat profusely as often as you can.

7. Massage. Schedule a massage each week if your time and budget permits.

8. Laugh. Try to do something every day that makes you laugh out loud. It changes the body chemistry for the better and releases stress.

9. Lubricate. Drink two tablespoons of olive oil every night before you go to bed.

10. Write. Keep a daily log of what you eat, what your incessant thoughts are about, how you are feeling, and how you slept the night before.

11. Record your progress photographically. Take a picture of yourself every day, from the same angle, at the same distance.

12. Eat a clove of garlic every day. Have it alone or thinly sliced and sandwiched between two thin apple slices.

➤

13. Read a book related to health and well-being, about the food system, or about the environment. Take this opportunity to educate yourself about what is going on today in your body. Understanding will make it more likely that you will want to maintain the results after you complete the program.

14. Express your artistic side. Dance, sing, play your instrument, paint, sculpt. Whatever it is that wets your whistle. This will activate your right brain and more strongly imprint this whole experience in that part of the brain, which is more involved with instincts. Far in the future, even if the thoughts of living Clean vanish, your instincts will be stronger than your thinking brain and will guide you to making the right choices for health.

distracted by a busy life that we reflexively reach for food when it's not actually needed. Or because we're uncomfortable having that body sensation and just want to get rid of it. Or we're just bored and looking for stimulation. After completing Clean, my patients often say they've learned to *be* with hunger instead of reactively killing it, which is a very powerful tool for life. When you crack this nut, you acquire the ability to take control over what you eat, when you eat, and how much of it you need to consume to feel your best.

THE CLEAN PLANNER

There is no one way to organize and accomplish Clean. Those who prefer to operate free of structure or planning can simply flip to the recipe section each day and improvise as they go, provided that ingredients are on hand. Others will benefit from writing a plan in advance, using the weekly chart provided for you on pages 192–193. You can download copies of this planner at www.cleanprogram.com. Planning will not only keep you focused and accountable for your actions but also will save you time. However you decide to proceed, please read the material in this section; it walks you through your first Clean program.

Before each week begins, pick out some recipes, being realistic, but as adventurous as possible. Get a sense of what ingredients you'll need and make a shopping list. Even if you don't stick to the exact recipe plan, you'll be well supplied. Fill out the planner, jotting down any supplements you plan to use as a reminder. Note any optional practices you want to include, including treatments or yoga or exercise classes outside the home. Jot down reminders of things you might forget about, like taking time to write. Put your chart on the fridge or somewhere you will see it easily.

Seven-Day Planner

SUNDAY	MONDAY	TUESDAY	WEDNESDAY
Breakfast	Breakfast	Breakfast	Breakfast
_____	_____	_____	_____
Lunch	Lunch	Lunch	Lunch
_____	_____	_____	_____
Dinner	Dinner	Dinner	Dinner
_____	_____	_____	_____
Supplements	Supplements	Supplements	Supplements
_____	_____	_____	_____
_____	_____	_____	_____
_____	_____	_____	_____
Appointments	Appointments	Appointments	Appointments
_____	_____	_____	_____
_____	_____	_____	_____
_____	_____	_____	_____

Checklist:

Checklist:	Checklist:	Checklist:	Checklist:
☐ 5-Min. Meditation	☐ 5-Min. Meditation	☐ 5-Min. Meditation	☐ 5-Min. Meditation
☐ Exercise	☐ Exercise	☐ Exercise	☐ Exercise
☐ Skin Brushing	☐ Skin Brushing	☐ Skin Brushing	☐ Skin Brushing
☐ Hot/Cold Plunge	☐ Hot/Cold Plunge	☐ Hot/Cold Plunge	☐ Hot/Cold Plunge
Reminders	Reminders	Reminders	Reminders
_____	_____	_____	_____
_____	_____	_____	_____
_____	_____	_____	_____
_____	_____	_____	_____

THURSDAY	FRIDAY	SATURDAY	SHOPPING
Breakfast	Breakfast	Breakfast	LIST

Lunch   Lunch   Lunch

Dinner   Dinner   Dinner

Supplements Supplements Supplements

Appointments Appointments Appointments

Checklist: **Checklist:** **Checklist:**
- ☐ 5-Min. Meditation ☐ 5-Min. Meditation ☐ 5-Min. Meditation
- ☐ Exercise ☐ Exercise ☐ Exercise
- ☐ Skin Brushing ☐ Skin Brushing ☐ Skin Brushing
- ☐ Hot/Cold Plunge ☐ Hot/Cold Plunge ☐ Hot/Cold Plunge

Reminders **Reminders** **Reminders**

Week 1

The first week of Clean is usually the most challenging because it involves the biggest changes. You are not only getting used to putting a different kind of food and drink in your body, you also have to get accustomed to preparing new meals and altering routines of how, where, and maybe with whom you eat. You may have to revisit the intentions you set and keep your inspiration up. Do whatever it takes—and get your rest. The first week is also when some people experience the symptoms of withdrawal from sugars, caffeine, and the chemicals in foods, especially if they didn't do a short Elimination Diet phase. Headaches, irritability, and other changes in mood and function are common in these first few days, and will pass soon.

Be ready for dealing with possible breakdowns in resolve. Have a sense of humor and acceptance about this whole process. It's not the end of the world if you waver for a moment, but a strong mental attitude will help you avoid breakdowns—and the wasted energy in worrying that comes with them.

One of my patients once asked me, in the middle of Week 1 of Clean, "I had some wine and some bread last night. Does that mean I ruined the whole program and should give up?"

I told him no. You took a step backward, but you did not ruin the whole thing. Just continue doing the program as if it had not happened, and take this opportunity to transform a breakdown into a breakthrough. The fact that you are interpreting what happened as a mistake stems from your desire for change, and this in itself is very positive! Hold on to that; don't guilt-trip yourself—guilt is a very toxic emotion in itself—or judge yourself. Just recommit to following the rest of the program with greater resolve. And if you want to make up for the one backward step, take two steps forward. Accelerate your cleanse a little by doing a day or two of only liquid meals.

Week 2

Now that you have gotten used to some new habits and to dealing with hunger, Week 2 is when much of the adaptation happens inside. It can be inspiring, or unsettling. Your body is adapting to a new state, reclaiming energy from digestion and starting some restoration work. If things were out of balance before, this shifting can feel awkward. Patterns can get disturbed (sleep, bowel movements, appetite, emotions). Use the information provided throughout this book to regulate what you need, but be open to things happening off your ordinary schedule and just go with the temporary changes. Accommodate your adapting body. (Meanwhile, don't overly accommodate other people if you can avoid it.) It can take ten days to two weeks to repair the average intestinal flora, meaning if you have not done a week of the Elimination Diet, you won't necessarily feel tremendous by Week 2 of the program. But change is happening.

BAD DREAMS

It's not unusual to have bad dreams at night or bad moods by day. What is getting dislodged and eliminated is not just the toxicity caused by chemicals but also the quantum toxins of stress and anxiety. Anytime we let the body unwind, it will throw off everything that has been clogging it, and that includes negative emotions and trauma. Be kind to yourself if this happens, know that it will pass, and try not to pay it forward to innocent bystanders at home or work. Don't judge any mood swings; don't overthink them. It may help to know the meditator's credo when it comes to this kind of quantum unwinding: "Better out than in."

HEADACHES

Another problem can be headaches. One patient told me, "I'm getting headaches—wouldn't it be better to take an Advil than to be distracted by them?" My answer was no. Do not take nonprescription medications during Clean. Ride out the headaches and they will go away just as they came. If the headaches are severe, you can take a nap, take valerian root (an herbal remedy), go for a walk or do some stretching exercises, take a bath, or do anything your instincts tell you may help, including massage or acupuncture. Medications such as Advil may improve the short-term situation, but your headaches will probably return even more strongly when the medication wears off. Headaches tend to disappear after the first few days of the program.

ENERGY SURGES

You may find, when you have done Clean for one or two weeks, that you feel so energetic that you are almost jittery. You can't sleep as easily or as long as normal and may feel the need to take a sleeping pill. I advise against this. You're starting to feel the surge of extra energy that has been liberated by reducing your food intake. It may take a little while for your body to know what to do with this extra energy. In the meantime, put it to good work. Go for a walk or a run, even in the middle of the night. Get some house cleaning done and reorganize your closets. Read a book or write those letters you should have written months ago. This is a temporary shifting in energy allocation and can even be fun. Soon, and at a natural pace, everything will fall into place and calm will return.

WEIGHT LOSS

Something else that is hard to predict is weight loss. You may find that you lose weight during the first ten days but then get stuck. You may wonder whether you are doing something wrong. Bear in mind that weight loss might occur in spurts during Clean. Don't worry. Make sure that you are having abundant bowel movements. There should be an increase in total daily amount compared to before the program started if you want to get the maximum possible effect. You can promote weight loss by increasing your daily exercise. This is also where you'll see the benefits of getting infrared saunas, massages, and colonics. Drink lots of water with fresh-squeezed lemon juice. To accelerate detoxification and weight loss, try consuming only liquid meals for a day or two more. Just take this day by day; see how it feels and monitor yourself. If you aren't getting enough food to support you in your daily life, you will know.

MUCOID PLAQUE

An aspect to detox programs that is frequently misunderstood is mucoid plaque. During an intensive cleanse such as a water or juice fast, there can be a sudden upturn in the amount of feces being eliminated which doesn't correlate with the amount of food that the individual is ingesting. People are often totally shocked: they have had nothing but juice for a week or more, have been eliminating daily, and suddenly, as their program hits top speed, they are dumping out lots of feces. Sometimes it is dark, almost tar-like, or it comes out as long ropes with the shape of colon foldings. Other times it is more like diarrhea.

This is the stuff of legend in the cleansing world. Many books will show you photographs of this matter, if you dare to look. The books, as well as many alternative healers, still (with the best of intentions) give information that is in my opinion, plain wrong. They claim that this dark matter is the debris of years of meals, especially meat, that has somehow gotten impacted on the mucosa or intestinal wall, and is finally getting released after multiple days of fasting. From my experience in both the cleansing and conventional medicine worlds, this legend is just not supported by scientific evidence. Here the technology of modern medicine is very useful in exposing the truth. Any gastroenterologist can tell you what they see in a colonoscopy (a process of looking at the colon wall using a scope, to check for disease). Their patients who have been given a strong laxative to dump the last one, two, or three days of waste in their intestines, have clean, pink intestinal walls. There is no sign of this mythic "years of debris" clinging to the intestines. Even in the sickest people whose mucosa shows the disease of chronic intestinal problems like ulcerative colitis, Crohn's disease, or cancer, there is no old stuck matter.

So what is all this old gunk that might come out (often to the person's great relief)? It is mucus that is finally getting dumped out of the cells and tissues, back into the blood circulation, and through the intestinal walls into the lumen of the intestine. The technical term for this is the "mucoid plaque." Because it's so sticky, it doesn't just fall into the intestines. It starts to accumulate on the intestinal walls as sweat does on your skin. Drop by drop, it builds up until suddenly, after seven to ten days of intensive fasting, there is a lot of it covering the intestinal walls, sticking things up. This can be a problem for someone who is cleansing or fasting without guidance. If the toxic matter isn't moved out with the help of strong fiber, excellent herbal laxatives that cause major elimination, and ideally, colonics, it can get reabsorbed and there is retox with the detox. The person might feel sick or even experience some kind of dysfunction in their tissues or organs.

This dramatic level of offloading won't happen with Clean's slightly slower detox process. But patients who are starting from a cleaner state, do often report some version of this "shedding" toward the end of their program, and feel immensely better as a result. Should this happen during your program, keep hydrated and be thankful for what you are losing. (And remember that wise saying, "Better out than in.")

For all these reasons, continuing past the second week is highly recommended. And if you do decide to finish the program after Week 2, it's important to remember that at this point you have established a delicate balance in the intestines. You are partway through the process of restoring intestinal integrity, so don't return immediately to sugar, alcohol, or the exact diet you had before you started Clean. Follow the tips in the next section for completing Clean. (And if you were considering stopping at the end of Week 2 but suspect that you can actually keep going, recommit and carry on!)

Week 3

As you start this final week, the end is in sight. You are two-thirds of the way through, so don't give up. At this point you will be in a good routine; keeping up your resolve isn't as hard because you have built a new set of habits. If you need motivation, ask your support system (your designated friend, family, or Clean partner) for help. Schedule a massage, take time for yoga, or do anything that is nurturing. Transformation can be hard, but know that the payoff for all your work is on the way: this week you start to reap the benefits. You feel the natural high that comes with detoxification; your skin glows, your eyes are whiter, your clothes are a little looser, and friends ask if you've just been on vacation (or had a face lift). Typically, the third week of Clean is when it hits you—this is how good you can feel at your age and stage in life. Just like the plant that has gotten nourished at the roots, you start to bloom, and healthy, shiny leaves and bright petals are the result. Let this be the inspiration to keep going through the full twenty-one days.

Kim, a twenty-eight-year-old architect, came to see me with one main complaint, a persistent, unrelenting cough. She coughed so much that it was affecting everything in her life, from her work to her sleep to her relationships. She had consulted with many doctors. She had even been seen by lung specialists and had undergone every imaging test that exists, from chest X-rays to CT scans, MRIs, and gallium scans. Nobody could find a clear problem. She was given special antibiotics that kill mystery bacteria known to cause a longstanding pneumonia that is marked by constant cough without fever or other symptoms. The coughing didn't stop. Next she was given anti-allergic medications. These didn't work. Then steroids were prescribed, which worked for a bit, until they stopped working. Her lung specialist wanted to increase the dosage and schedule a bronchoscopy—an invasive procedure that involves inserting a scope down a person's throat and into the lungs. In a desperate attempt to avoid the bronchoscopy, Kim came to see me. After a three-week cleanse her cough had completely disappeared. But something else happened that blew my mind. She did not need her reading glasses anymore, a symptom that she had not even mentioned because she thought of it as just part of getting older—most of the adults in her family wear glasses, and they all had to start wearing them early in life. I still scratch my head over Kim's recovery and its welcome side effect. Did the restored intestinal flora and the energy recaptured by the detox allow her body to finally heal? Did she lose mucus from the eye area, aiding her eyesight? In any case, obstacles were clearly removed, lacking ingredients were added, and Kim's innate natural intelligence did the rest. When given a chance, even the most fatigued body wants to find its way back to balance.

CHAPTER EIGHT

After the Cleanse

Congratulations on completing Clean. By now you are probably having a very different experience of your body than before Clean. If you did not get all the results you were hoping for, it's perfectly fine and safe to continue with the program for a few days or even a week or two longer. Some patients of mine have even stayed on it for several months. In fact, though you'd probably need a slight increase in quantity of food, you could safely keep on eating this way for the rest of your life, since the way you've been eating during the program is much closer to the way nature intended you to eat. True, nature doesn't come with a blender, but the ingredients and the proportions of raw to cooked foods you have gotten used to have put you more in line with the way we, and all the other animals on the planet, were intended to eat. In an age of processed, devitalized food and tired, overburdened bodies, this can only be a good thing.

There are different ways to return to your previous style of life. You could finish Clean cold turkey on day 22, and pick up the same eating habits you had before you began. But if you were feeling slower and looking older before Clean—which is what most of my own patients report—do you really want to do that?

In my experience, almost nobody wants to go back to feeling the way they did before. Some people have such a profound transformation that even years later they have held on to enough of what they've learned to continue to enjoy the benefits. Others get a huge boost during the three weeks itself, but in the months afterward find that old habits, and the symptoms of toxicity, return because life gets busy and full of distractions again. Still others end the program only to return the very next day to the exact same eating and drinking habits they had before, inadvertently eroding some of the improvements to their inner environments. Which of these three scenarios ends up applying to you depends on how you transition out of the program and what you do to maintain its benefits, so read this chapter carefully.

COMPLETING CLEAN

You may be impatient to return to regular meals. Or you might feel that at this point a few more days of Clean would be a cinch. In either case, please transition out of Clean gradually. Start by going to one liquid meal and two solid meals a day, continuing to choose meals from the Clean recipes or the Elimination Diet. Many of my patients never abandon this equation. The majority of them prefer to have the liquid meal for breakfast. It's quick and easy to prepare and gives a lighter but still nourishing start to the day. You can use the Clean smoothie and juice recipes or be creative and invent some yourself. After a few days of doing this, return to three solid-food meals a day if you like—but *continue to adhere to the Elimination Diet rules.*

Do not yet return to your pre-Clean diet. You have a unique opportunity, one that most people today never get. For several weeks you've avoided all the foods known to cause food allergies, food sensitivities, and digestive strain. You've created a clean canvas on which to do some life-changing research. With a little patience and discipline, you can investigate what thousands of people pay huge amounts of money to do, and find out which foods disturb your body and might cause some of the symptoms you've gotten used to shouldering.

As you have discovered, mild to severe reactions against certain foods are commonplace. Remember, the activity may be happening far below the surface and not felt in obvious ways beyond fatigue or dullness. Or it may be experienced as full-blown allergic attacks. Two people standing next to each other will have vastly different responses to the same irritant and it's impossible to predict who will have which response. But whether your response is mild or extreme, if you want to find the triggers, typically you have to choose between two diagnostic tools. The first is a laboratory blood test called an antibody profile. This scans a blood sample for antibodies to a wide variety of foods, both the kinds of antibodies that might cause full-blown allergic reactions and those that trigger subtler, more delayed food sensitivity responses. I offer these tests to patients who have the money or the desire to see results on paper, usually to confirm what they've found out through completing Clean and doing the detective work that you are about to do. However, the truth is that blood tests are not totally reliable. They sometimes fail to detect food allergies. Sometimes the tests cross-react with other antibodies and get the causes of the allergy confused. These tests don't do a good job of detecting the lower-grade irritants that cause hidden food sensitivities.

Likewise, the skin tests performed by allergy specialists are time consuming and complicated, involving many repeat visits to the doctor. They are not completely accurate, either, and they come with a potentially huge downside: once you are told you are allergic to a certain food, you will never freely enjoy it again, even if the diagnosis was incorrect.

Clean gives you the opportunity to be your own detective. Freed from processing anything potentially irritating, your system has balanced itself and returned to its optimal conditions for healthy functioning. You can use a low-tech and cost-free method to determine your food sensitivities, one that is more accurate than any other available methods. It only takes a little commitment and some observation.

IDENTIFYING YOUR TOXIC TRIGGERS

Two to three days after finishing the Clean program, or whenever you have transitioned to three solid meals a day, introduce one type of food from the Elimination Diet's "exclude" list into your daily meals. Perhaps it is wheat or one of the other gluten grains. Have a sandwich at lunch or have a bagel for breakfast. If you want to start with milk, have a latte, some yogurt, or cheese. You don't need to have a whole loaf of bread or a quart of milk; a moderate serving of the food in question will do. Observe and feel what happens over the next twenty-four hours. It is helpful to record comments in your Clean log for each food you introduce. Notice the following:

How do you feel immediately after eating it? Are there any sensations in your belly?

Does anything happen shortly after you eat it, such as a runny nose or mucus in the throat (typical of milk), or fatigue, bloating, or headache (typical of wheat)?

How are your energy levels? A bowl of wheat pasta at night, for example, may make you feel very tired either immediately after eating it or on waking up the next morning.

How are your bowel movements the next day? As frequent and as easy to eliminate as they were during Clean, or are they now altered?

How did you sleep that night? Was it a heavier sleep, or were you disturbed?

How does your skin look, and how are your emotions the following day?

Any noticeable change in your physical or mental experience is an indication that you might be sensitive or fully allergic to that food. To make this process even more accurate, eat the same food the next day and see if it provokes a reaction. (The second day the reaction may be slightly milder as the contrast is less pronounced.) Again, notice what happens for a full day after eating the food. It is likely that some of the foods from the list will reveal themselves to you as toxic triggers: foods that are either mildly disturbing to your natural balance or actually allergenic.

Repeat the same process with every item of the "no" foods that you really like or miss. The most common foods my patients find to be toxic triggers include these, now familiar to you: Dairy (predominantly cow's milk and products made from it); eggs; wheat and gluten-containing grains such as rye and barley; fatty red meat; soy products; corn (in this instance, corn tortillas and corn chips could be your testing food), and chocolate.

If you have a severe allergy to one of these foods it will be quite obvious to you. Gluten sensitivity is a prime example. Some people have such a bad reaction to gluten, the protein in wheat, barley, and rye, that it causes a cluster of extreme symptoms known as celiac disease, which severely limits nutrient absorption in the small intestine, with devastating consequences. But many others have a subtler reaction to the gluten that goes undiagnosed, because they assume that their chronic but non-urgent conditions must be related to other things, like being tired and run down from life or having a more sensitive constitution than normal. They may have gotten used to suffering these conditions for years, like being fatigued, frequently feeling they're on the verge of catching a cold, having headaches, or regularly having constipation or diarrhea. Doing this investigation into irritants can be a revelation: they are able to identify their breakfast muffin or lunchtime penne pasta as a trigger of these symptoms, and they realize they are best off avoiding wheat and other gluten-containing grains entirely.

The effects of alcohol, caffeine (especially coffee), and sugar will also now be "louder." With your clean Clean canvas, you'll get a sense of their true impact on your particular constitution. If you still desire them, reintroduce them one at a time, consuming them in reasonable amounts, and notice the effects on your body, your energy levels throughout the day, and your mental outlook. Take some notes to serve as your evidence later about how these things affect you when you are in your cleanest state. There is no need to be a purist for the rest of your life if you enjoy wine, beer, cheesecake, or chocolate. Have them, and enjoy them—there's nothing worse for digestion than guilt—and bring your awareness fully to the present moment with each bite or sip. Eating in this very conscious way, you might find that the larger amounts you used to consume have a stronger impact than you noticed before and that much smaller amounts please you. Buying smaller amounts of higher-quality products always helps.

If your reaction to any of the foods you test is mild but still noticeable (slight fatigue, constipation, blue mood) you might not want to eliminate it forever, but you will still benefit from reducing the frequency of exposure to it. Following a "rotation diet" is a simple way to avoid the negative consequences of mild to moderate food allergies and sensitivities. Rotate your choice of foods so that you don't eat the irritating ones more than once every four days.

This process of investigating your toxic triggers may sound complicated at first. It is not. In fact, it's a breeze compared to what you just accomplished with Clean, and the potential for discovering how to maintain the benefits you got during the program and avoid returning to old symptoms is priceless.

Rich came to my office with complaints of severe irritable bowel syndrome. He had it so badly that he was starting to see a decline in his effectiveness at work, where his attacks of diarrhea, often with cramping, hit him hardest. Most of all, his quality of life was greatly affected. He thought that since the attacks were worse at work than at home on the weekends, it was most likely linked to his sometimes stressful job. I asked Rich to do Clean. To his surprise, the symptoms completely resolved as if by magic, even during the most stressful of days. He continued to follow the Elimination Diet for several weeks, until he allowed himself to eat from the list of "no" foods again. During this detective work we found the answer to his problem, loud and clear. What Rich most missed from his forbidden foods was the egg salad sandwich that was his standard workday lunch. Two hours after once again eating his beloved egg salad, the diarrhea he got was so violent that we were left no doubt: eggs were his trigger. Rich had spent fifteen years getting tested by different doctors in an effort to clear his bowel syndrome. None of the blood tests performed for food allergies had ever detected the egg allergy. It took doing his own investigation to reveal the answer. Four years since that last sandwich, Rich remains symptom-free.

STAYING CLEAN: THE MONTHS TO COME

Preparation is important before you do the Clean program and maintenance is critical afterward. What you've just accomplished during your three weeks is monumental. You restored your body to a more natural state. You gave the body back its natural ability to defend itself, restore itself, heal and even rejuvenate. By clearing out some of the toxic overload and restoring nutrients, you have literally cleared out some of the obstacles and restored many of the lacks getting in the way of healthy functioning. You are experiencing the benefits already in the way you look, feel, think, and sleep, and in your reduced vulnerability to common sicknesses. Some old ideas have been turned on their heads. For example, one accepted belief is that bacteria and viruses attack you and make you toxic and ill. This is like saying the mice and roaches make the trash can full—a crude analogy, but an apt one. The real reason roaches and mice hang out in the trash can is because garbage is there attracting them. Likewise, bacteria and viruses will land and thrive in bodies that are already toxic. You have just emptied your trash and scrubbed the can itself clean. The scavengers will find you very boring—they'll go straight to your neighbor's in search of their meal.

Furthermore, you have started to create the kind of inner environment that fends off not only bad bacteria and viruses but also the many other diseases and sicknesses of modern civilization that bedevil so many

Americans as they get older. Conserve and take care of this environment, and they need never find their way to your door.

Of course you want to stay this way. You want to get through seasonal changes without allergies, avoid long winter colds, maintain a leaner body, retain bright, glowing skin, keep your digestion functioning well, continue to sleep calmly, and stay energized through the day.

This is more than possible. This state of well-being is resilient. It is natural to you. And therefore it is quite self-sustaining when you support it with maintenance and periodic follow-ups. This is basic common sense. If you constructed a fantastic new building, it would be foolish to not maintain it. If you invested in a new car, you'd maintain it just as the user's manual instructs, to keep it running well over the months and years to come. For some reason, we're more resistant to this idea when it comes to our health. It's easier and more convenient to let things go a little and then look for the next fix-it solution when systems and organs start to degenerate. The "magic bullet" approach is rampant in American culture today. Ignore things until they get intolerable, and then hunt out that diet, supplement, surgery, or natural therapy that promises to reverse it all tomorrow. Magazines, movies, and TV shows support this approach overwhelmingly. Magazine covers feature pictures of celebrities and headlines about what they did to look ten years younger—which becomes the next fad of the moment. But what if we saw that celebrity a few months or years later? Often they've backslid from that high state of health back to where they were before, or worse. Usually lack of maintenance is the cause. They did the kick-start without any follow-up.

Clean will give you great results, but don't expect it to be your magic bullet; see it as a profound and well-deserved jumpstart to a more balanced way of living. Once you start, it's up to you to maintain the balance if you want to maintain the benefits. Use some of the principles you've already been practicing to build a system of eating and living that you can sustain on a daily basis.

I take pains to assure patients that this approach is different from signing up for a whole lifestyle make-over. Nobody has to eat a set way from now on, exercise the exact same way as the rest of the herd, or have a totally green eco-home and office. In all these areas do what works best for you according to your natural interest and enthusiasm, enjoy your life, and keep evolving by taking steps forward. You should find making any kind of change a little easier now that you can hear more clearly which habits or foods make you function better, and which ones make you stuck, drained, or toxic. This is how long-term radiant well-being is built. It comes from you knowing your needs best. There's an avalanche of wellness information out there to guide and inspire you.

Western medicine is slowly waking up to how the "one size fits all" approach to medicine is failing us. New data reveal that wonder drugs do not do wonderful things for all patients, because we all vary in our genetic predispositions. A variation in genes may leave one person without the enzyme needed to eliminate a certain drug and may cause a harmful high concentration of the drug in the blood. Researchers are now finding that most drugs, no matter what the disease, work for only half the patients for whom they are prescribed. As a result of the severe wastage of these drugs—literally billions of dollars' worth—and to some extent because of concerns for the possible damage done by unwisely prescribed drugs, a new era of "personalized medicine" is definitely on the horizon in our allopathic (drug-based) health-care system. In this coming era, diagnostic technologies that are still slightly on the fringes—such as doing tests to screen for genetic tendencies before prescribing expensive drugs, or testing for vitamin D levels—will become much more common.

Eastern traditions of health care have always known that one size can't fit all. It's all personalized. A doctor will first advise some basic, commonsense groundwork that is good for everyone to do, such as clearing out toxins and bringing the inner environment back to balance, just as you have done with Clean. This process gets the ball rolling and starts the healing. If it's not enough to solve everything, then the practitioner evaluates individual constitution, personality, and preferences to determine the right kind of treatment. To give you an idea of the difference between the approaches, a Western doctor might diagnose ten patients with similar symptoms as having the same disease, and give them the exact same treatment. The Chinese medicine doctor may see the same patients and have as many as seven different diagnoses for the similar symptoms. She or he will consequently prescribe a different treatment for each patient, appropriate to each one's unique needs.

The Eastern and Western approaches are combined in integrative, or open-minded, medicine. When advising patients on how to maintain themselves Clean and healthy, I recommend a few general "foundational" tools—the Clean maintenance plan—that everyone living the modern lifestyle in busy cities can use to maintain the benefits and support the conditions for healing. The Clean maintenance plan is not a strict regime, but instead is a way to draw attention to four important areas that, if you keep an eye on them, will ensure that you feel and look as good as you can for your age and stage of life.

What patients do on top of this baseline will inevitably vary from person to person, as their goals, hopes, specific health challenges, age, and body types differ so widely. The common theme that unites everyone after doing their first Clean program is that they've experienced in their own bodies how much they can author their own state of well-being. They have realized the most "personalized medicine" of all because they've touched the power they have to truly heal themselves.

Keep this in mind as you move forward. There are thousands of theories about diet, lifestyle, and stress management out there, and everyone has her own opinion on how you should live. Take in as much or as little of that as you like; but first and foremost keep your foundation solid by maintaining what you've just achieved through the Clean Program.

Like a house with four pillars, the maintenance plan focuses on four areas:

1. Eat Clean: How to eat after Clean
2. Detox periodically: How often and when to Clean in the future

3. Reduce exposure to toxins: Realistic steps to Clean your immediate environment of toxins as best you can, including the quantum toxicity of stress

4. Maintain a Clean bill of health: Working in partnership with a doctor to continue to evolve your health and avoid prescription medications, medical interventions, and disease.

1. EAT CLEAN

The first question people have upon returning to their regular routine is almost always "What do I eat now?" There are so many books about the perfect diet for humans that it makes everyone dizzy. People often decide that one or the other theory makes sense and launch themselves into that lifestyle, only to discover it ends up making them sick. I have personally tried many different plans over the years, for different reasons, from athletic training to losing that chubbiness I wrote of earlier. What I learned is that most of them do work for a specific purpose. Some plans quickly make you lean, others maximize your muscle mass, and still others make you lose weight in a dramatic, and not so appealing, fashion. My summation, however, is that when weight loss is the only focus of diet, any patient is bound to end up far from healthy and vibrant.

The Eat Clean Maintenance Checklist

Continue to include the habits you began during your three-week detox program for ongoing good health. In addition to lowering your intake of the foods you found to be irritating, do the following:

- Eat more alkaline than acidic foods (eat lots of vegetables). Lower your intake of the mucus-forming foods (dairy, sugar, wheat, white rice).
- Eat more organic produce, more hormone- and antibiotic-free animal products and meats, and seek out products that have not been genetically modified.
- Include plenty of the fresh, whole foods containing the key nutrients for health and detoxification in your diet every week.
- Eat at least 51 percent or more of your food raw (vegetables, fruits, seeds, nuts, unprocessed oils.
- Support thriving good bacteria in your intestinal tract with plenty of fiber, good-quality saturated fats, foods with naturally occurring probiotics (raw and unprocessed sauerkraut, organic kefir, kombucha, kimchee). Avoid feeding the bad bacteria. Avoid anything with

Instead of deciding which diet book is right, I look at the book of nature. This is basically the protocol you have been following in Clean, in a slightly modified way. When we return to what nature originally designed for us, and eat closer to what every other animal eats, this alone begins to heal us. This very simple preservatives; reduce sugar, wheat, and refined grains; avoid dairy products and alcohol. Lower your stress levels and avoid prescription drugs and over-the-counter medications when possible.

- Follow an anti-inflammatory diet filled with nature's anti-inflammatories and take fish oil, or flaxseed and hemp oils if you are vegetarian.

- Support your local farmers' market or local farmers; locally grown foods have more nutrition, because they're picked closer to their end-use locale and thus can be picked when they are ripe.

- "Eat what you are." Maintain a calm state of mind, an active body, and a clean intestine and you won't set up the conditions for cravings. Fuel yourself with what will best serve the person you want to be.

- Treat the planet's animals well. Eat with awareness of your food's impact on the whole. As the current tidal wave of movies such as *The Future of Food* explain well and simply, the choices you make when buying food have effects more far-reaching than their effect on your body and well-being.

concept is radical if you're used to the idea that dominates the American psyche: that the sole objective of healthy eating should be weight loss.

The debate over which dietary plan is optimal for humans has become an obsession centering on calories and pounds, one that has taken society on a roller-coaster ride of overnight fads (described in an earlier chapter) with more than a few damaging consequences. Having witnessed how countless patients, including myself, lose their depression after good intestinal conditions are restored, there is no doubt in my mind of the connection. If you are a scientist or physician, then forgive the crude oversimplification of a complex subject. Yet it's important to consider this question, both literally, through an understanding of metabolic function, and philosophically. What have we done by losing our ability to listen to our real needs and follow our instincts, by surrendering to market-driven eating instead? How are we causing our own toxicity by veering so far from natural patterns?

Looking at the experiences of my patients at both Lenox Hill Hospital and the Eleven Eleven Wellness Center, I have begun to believe that the current rise in chronic diseases such as heart disease, cancer, and depression is tightly linked to the high-protein madness that puts no limits on the consumption of meat. The diet that so many people follow to get skinnier just might be one of the biggest factors in their toxicity.

This raises the question of whether eating animal products is healthy or unhealthy. Personally, I think it almost requires a doctorate in nutrition to be a healthy vegetarian. To my mind, if transitioning to a vegetarian diet appeals to someone for health, moral, or ecological reasons, it should be a goal to work toward in stages, guided by an expert or at the very least, wise books like Dr. Cousens's.

If all this raises more questions about how to eat than it answers, then that's all to the good. I prefer not to present a single, definitive answer (which I don't have to offer) but instead to set you on your own path to creating the diet that works best for your present understanding, interest, time commitment, financial resources, and geographical location, among other factors. What I do state without any reservations is that maintaining a Clean way of eating as the foundation of your diet to as great an extent as possible will prove highly beneficial—and possibly life saving—in the months and years to come.

2. DETOX PERIODICALLY

The next most common question post-Clean is "When do I cleanse again?" How often and how long you do cleanses and detoxification programs will depend on how clean your diet and lifestyle stay and what kind of results you're looking for. By now it's clear to you that modern lifestyles and big cities make it impossible to completely avoid toxicity. Clean has shown you how inner pollution needs to be cleared out, even if you can't see it as clearly as the grime on your skin. As a general rule, most people who are not suffering from any diseases or symptoms, feel consistently well, and want to stay that way, will benefit from doing the full Clean program once a year. Should you want to improve your state more significantly because you have lingering symptoms, do it every six months. Doing your full three-week program on an annual or biannual schedule is enough for most people. Repeat it too often, and the possible side effect is boredom. Too seldom, and you may find the enthusiasm dampens.

As part of a maintenance program, I use Clean myself and prescribe it to patients in two main ways: to maintain and improve upon the condition created by the last full-length cleanse; and as a tool to get back on the path right away if old eating and drinking habits creep back or associated symptoms flare up again. Here are two common scenarios that occur in people's lives post-Clean.

You've been doing pretty well maintaining a healthy diet, but during a party or holiday weekend, you let go a little. You feel bloated and sluggish. Make the next day a juice fast. Make sure you have abundant bowel movements, using herbal laxatives if necessary. If you don't bounce back immediately, repeat this the next day, or shift to one solid meal and two liquid ones. Play with it; be creative, and discover what works for you.

You've had a tough few weeks or months, and slowly the comfort foods and drinks have crept back in. You're getting puffy again and your spirits are lower than normal. Use Clean as a tool for re-centering yourself. Do one week, two weeks, or even just the Elimination Diet on its own, for as long as you need to clear out the gunk. The first time you do Clean, it is a jumpstart to a whole new way of life. After that, it becomes a signpost on your lifelong path, pointing you back to your goals. After a short derailment (a few weeks of eating toxic foods or being under great stress), do a short version of the program. If you wandered far off the road for several months of toxification, do a full Clean program.

Everyone can juice for one day a week. Your digestive system and bowels work hard six days a week; give them a rest on the seventh day. It's a biblical-sounding idea, like respecting the sabbath with your body. A day of digestive rest is not only calming to the spirit, it supports you in staying "caught up" with cleaning duties all year long. Weekly fasts have a cumulative effect: Four days of fasting a month becomes fifty-two days of fasting a year, which becomes a full year of fasting every seven years! Consider what

332 • ALEJANDRO JUNGER, M.D.

happens when agriculturists follow this pattern: After six years of cultivation, in the seventh year they typically rest their soil by leaving it fallow to recover for a full year. Nutrients are restored and life-giving energy is literally rebuilt into the ground. If you take care of your body with a similar level of attention, you will flourish too.

3. REDUCE EXPOSURE TO TOXINS: CREATING A CLEANER LIFESTYLE

Consider all the ways you're exposed to unnecessary stressors, and make the following changes over the next twelve months. These are the most important modifications you can do in a toxic world.

- Replace household cleaning and any personal products filled with unnecessary chemicals with natural ones.
- Invest in a water filtration system. William Wendling is a water expert I work with in Los Angeles. His systems are affordable and his service is timely and dependable. He ships his filters around the country and takes consultations for coaching you on acquiring a system that fits your needs and lifestyle. Visit www.oxygenozone.com for more information.

- Invest in an air filtration system. Room units or, better yet, entire household systems are well worth the investment. Please see William Wendling's Web site for more information.

- Cultivate an ongoing meditation practice—or whatever practice you think will provide the tools for avoiding quantum toxicity and encourage your own transformation. This could be a martial art, it could be working with a personal guide, or something very different.

- Become conscious of the amount of unnecessary information (excess media, news, entertainment you aren't even that interested in) and communication that may be in your life. Reduce whatever is superfluous, and recapture some of the attention that is lost this way each day.

- Boost your exercise and commit to a regular routine. Science is showing us with exciting new research how challenging workouts correlate with giant health benefits, so make a point to put this on your Wellness Plan.

- Get more sun, fill up on vitamin D, and everything else that is free if you only make time for it: friends, laughter, nature, and pleasure in its fullest sense.

4. MAINTAIN A CLEAN BILL OF HEALTH WITH A PARTNER IN HEALTH

Maintaining yourself Clean can primarily be done by you, on your own. But you want to have a like-minded partner at certain times and for specific needs. That partner is an open-minded doctor.

Working with a professional who understands and appreciates what you are building through diet, detoxing, and offloading stress is invaluable. Your current doctor may be an excellent ally—there is no need to fire her if, for example, you are concerned that she hasn't brought up nutrition and detoxification. Maybe you can start the conversation. Be critical and ask questions if you have the right partner. We're in the middle of a big shift in health care; there is a global movement redirecting medical professionals toward a more holistic approach. You want to be guided by a doctor who is at least open to exploring this territory. Even better, find a doctor who already practices medicine in an integrative way. For this, I recommend looking for practitioners who have studied Functional Medicine (find them at www.functional medicine.org). Whether meeting a new doctor or broaching the subject with your existing provider, interview her as if she were applying for the most important job in the world, taking care of you. Look into her eyes and see if she is present with you. Watch if she listens and is willing to rethink your treatment when the current approach is not working. Feel the atmosphere in the office. How does she relate to her nurses, technicians, and receptionist? Does it *feel* well in there? Or does it feel tired and drained? How did she respond when you told her about Clean? Now that you are more trained to listening in to your body and your instincts, you have the sensitivity to be the driver of your health. Take the wheel.

Of course, to get where you want to go you need a map. This is why you should have a simple checklist of goals you want to achieve in the year following your first detox program. Clean was your jumpstart; now ask the next set of questions: Do you need to lose weight? Do you want to transition off medications and regulate or improve conditions naturally? Do you want to get stronger to prevent osteoporosis, or maybe to look even better? Everyone has their own list, which can include simple concerns (clear up bad skin entirely; lose final fifteen pounds) or more involved ones (find a natural alternative to arthritis drugs that works for you; prepare for pregnancy). If you truly want to change, then all these things should be clear-cut goals that you have written down and can look at; they need to be things you tell your doctor about and work together to achieve.

They should be written on your calendar along with dates indicating when you hope to have achieved them, just as you did with your Clean program.

Wellness Coordinators and Coaches

To keep businesses running smoothly, we have CEOs, COOs, CFOs, presidents, vice presidents, executives, secretaries, assistants, receptionists—a whole army of people to initiate and then keep track of everything that has to be done to keep a business running smoothly. It is not a crazy idea, if you can afford, it to have a wellness coordinator. Someone who will meet with you periodically, review your goals, analyze where you might have failed in meeting them, and explore why. This person will help you reinforce your plan for success, keep your appointments, research the doctors you are referred to and the treatments that are prescribed for you.

It's amazing to see how my patients' efficiency skyrockets when they work with a wellness coordinator. When they come to my office they are now armed with all their previous tests organized in chronological order, saving time and avoiding repetition of expensive tests. They are more prepared mentally and stay on the program of building health with more ease. If you have some big goals for your own Wellness Plan, working with a wellness coordinator or coach may be a sound investment. This is not a very developed field. Maybe you can train your current assistant to include this as part of his or her job. Or simply find a person with the necessary qualities. I would look for a smart, curious, motivated, and organized person whom I feel a certain chemistry of inspiration. Be creative. Invent what works for you.

Blood Tests: Finding Your Blood Levels of Important Elements

Western medicine offers certain tools that will help you maintain and improve upon the benefits you get from Clean. Take advantage of them, and they may be priceless in helping you avoid unnecessary suffering. As a cardiologist I value blood tests for giving early insight into obstacles and lacks that might exist in the patient's body, conditions that if not corrected could tip them off balance and sow the seeds of coronary artery disease. When imbalances are caught early, changes in diet, exercise, supplements, and a Clean detoxification program can very often shift the balance back, as you've read throughout this book.

If this is so, why then is it still the case that a patient with a "normal" annual blood test can drop dead from a heart attack days after having the test? Why are so many people on statin drugs and heart medication as precautionary measures? Sometimes it's because they and their doctors aren't gathering all the information early enough that they could gather. Almost every doctor today, cardiologist or not, has tests done for cholesterol levels. But there are a few other basic blood tests that, when done yearly as part of your maintenance plan, can give you a hint of a heart attack in the making. Get your doctor to administer the following tests. A good doctor schooled in integrative health care will use the information from them to guide you to your goal of staying Clean, healthy, and youthful in a toxic world.

Inflammatory Markers. C-reactive protein (CRP) is a protein produced in the liver that is a marker of inflammation. When CRP levels are elevated it means your inflammatory system is turned "on," making you a candidate not only for heart disease but also for all the other conditions now linked to inflammation. Work with your doctor to figure out why inflammation is turned on: Is it from nutritional deficiencies, a hidden infection (such as parasites), or another insult somewhere in the body? The investigation you will do together will be priceless. Other markers of inflammation are ESR (erythrocyte sedimentation rate), blood insulin levels (insulin is a pro-inflammatory hormone), and fibrinogen (where inflammation and blood clotting systems meet, which means both clotting and inflammation use the same molecules).

AA/EPA Ratio. This is a more sophisticated marker of systemic inflammation than the CRP test, detecting inflammation at an even subtler level. It is the true marker of silent inflammation. The higher the ratio, the greater the amount of silent inflammation you have. If it is greater than 10, you have inflammation. A good ratio would be 3, and the ideal ratio is about 1.5. The average American score today is 11, and for those who already have developed inflammatory diseases it can be over 20. A higher ratio indicates that you are at risk of aging faster and losing health quicker.

Remember that inflammation is one of the body's necessary and potentially life-saving functions. The problem is when it occurs for no apparent reason because the balance between pro-inflammation and anti-inflammation is lost. Too much anti-inflammation can be as bad as too little. If the AA-to-EPA ratio is too low—for example, 0.7— you will be more prone to infections and you might not be able to mount an appropriate inflammatory response when you need to. (You can get this test through Nutrasource Diagnostics Inc.; 877-557-7722 or 519-827-8129.)

Lipoprotein (a). This type of fat is actually thought to be worse than LDL, the so-called "bad" cholesterol, and is associated with a sevenfold incidence of coronary disease. Statin drugs don't touch it, nor does exercise. Niacin works, but not always. When I find it elevated on my patients I order a CT angiogram for them.

Uric Acid. A waste product produced mainly as a byproduct of the processing of animal proteins, uric acid is toxic and causes gout (inflammation in the joints) as well as corrosion of arteries, increasing chances of arterial plaque deposit.

Vitamin D. More and more evidence links a deficiency of vitamin D with heart disease and also depression, osteoporosis, and cancer. Humans today protect themselves from the sun so much that they have become a species depleted of vitamin D. The consequences have been devastating. Early detection of low levels will help you modify your diet, take supplements if necessary, and get more sun.

Homocysteine. Homocysteine is an amino acid that is a waste product of the processing of proteins that is toxic when not effectively cleared by the liver. High levels in the blood plasma predispose people to coronary artery disease, Alzheimer's disease, and, in younger women, premature birth and other problems of the reproductive system. High levels usually respond to detoxification programs and supplementation with vitamin B complex.

Thyroid Function. Most doctors order tests for the thyroid hormones TSH (thyroid-stimulating hormone) and T4 (thyroxine), but Free T3 is the active thyroid hormone that needs to be checked. When T4 is converted to T3 and then to Free T3 and thus activated, our body needs certain vitamins and minerals to do it. Supplementing with these boosts thyroid activity and therefore metabolism and is often enough to correct mild clinical presentations of low thyroid activity.

Thyroglobulin Antibodies. Autoimmunity generated by gluten can have subtle expressions, such as the creation of antibodies against proteins of your thyroid system, called thyroglobulins. Catching high levels of these early can prevent future bigger problems.

The disruption of the intestinal lining exposes the GALT to antigens that should have been filtered out; many allergic reactions are generated this way. Gluten, a protein that appears in wheat and other grains, can generate an immune response, known as celiac disease. When severe, it can be fatal.

Iodine Levels. Iodine is what the thyroid gland uses to manufacture its products, thyroid hormones. Our food supply is lacking in adequate iodine. When lack of iodine is severe, we develop goiter, but there is growing evidence that milder iodine deficiencies are associated with heart disease, among other things. If you have thyroid abnormalities or symptoms you suspect have to do with your thyroid, ask your doctor to order an iodine absorption test (Doctor's Data is a laboratory that can provide you with the kit; contact them via their Web site www.doctorsdata.com).

Mercury and Other Heavy Metals. Mercury toxicity is called "the great mimicker" because it can show up as many different diseases, from psychiatric problems and cancers to autoimmune diseases. When your symptoms are not that clear, or do not seem to get better despite great efforts, or when you suspect exposure to heavy metals (you have consumed a lot of tuna or other mercury-laden fish or you have silver amalgam dental fillings), have your doctor test you for it. Blood mercury and hair analysis have their uses, but are not the way to determine if you are mercury toxic. The only reliable test is a twenty-four-hour Urine Challenge Test using a chelating agent such as DMSA. Metametrix or Doctors Data are the labs I use.

Organic Acid Test. Available from Metametrix. Allows you to tailor a supplement regimen specific to you, as opposed to taking whatever supplement is making the news (which may or may not be good for you).

A Personalized Supplement Regime

Design a supplement regimen tailored specifically for your needs, instead of blindly taking every vitamin or other supplement that happens to be making the news. The Organic Acid test by Metametrix in combination with simple blood levels of magnesium, zinc, selenium, Vitamin D and the B vitamins will give lots of information in order to do this.

YOUR CLEAN WELLNESS PLAN AT A GLANCE

Your list of goals for the next year may include some or all of the following. Add your own goals to the list.

1. Find an open-minded doctor.
2. Eat Clean: eat organic food, nothing processed, 51 percent raw, avoid chemicals, buy food at your local farmers' market.
3. Install water filters and air filters at home.
4. Do the Clean program periodically. Fast every night for twelve hours. Juice for one day a week, for five days with every change of season; and for one week to ten days a year. Or do some research and find the plan that resonates with you. More and more plans for detox are being talked about everywhere. Explore them.

5. Keep blood and inner environment alkaline. Periodically measure acidity by using pH strips on saliva.

6. Exercise.

7. Meditate.

8. Get body work (massage, chiropractic, reflexology, osteopathy, cranio-sacral therapy).

9. Do stretching, yoga, or Pilates.

10. Express creativity.

11. Rest and sleep.

12. Spend time with loved ones.

13. Establish a custom-tailored supplement regimen.

14. Get blood tests and other tests once a year.

15. Read and learn about health and wellness.

16. Find a wellness coordinator.

CHAPTER NINE

Cardiovascular Disease and Toxicity

As a cardiologist I was trained to treat heart attacks and their complications. Those critical moments that require fast thinking, smart decisions, and a little luck were what attracted me to becoming a cardiologist in the first place. The result of saving a life is evident immediately, and the feeling of doing it is right up there with the other greatest feelings in life. Western medicine has amazing technology to open the arteries and restore blood flow to the heart muscle. Angiograms, angioplasties, and stents have proved invaluable in those life and death situations.

Yet all the training cardiologists get and all the advances in technology are not enough. Heart disease is still the number one killer in the United States. We have not been able to significantly reduce its impact.

What are we missing?

America has been looking for the culprit forever. As it turns out, we found many culprits. We call them "risk factors." The more of these you have, the more likely you are to develop blockages in your coronary arteries and suffer a possible subsequent heart attack.

The classic risk factors are diabetes, smoking, high blood pressure, family history of heart attacks or genetic predisposition, and high cholesterol.

Then there are other risk factors that are not so well known:

- High uric acid level. Uric acid is a waste product that irritates the arteries and promotes heart disease. Acidity in general exacerbates heart disease.
- High lipoprotein (a) level. Lipoprotein (a) is another kind of fat in blood; it is associated in a stronger way with the likelihood of blocked arteries than LDL, the classic "bad cholesterol" fat most people are familiar with.
- High homocysteine level. Homocysteine is a waste product of the processing of certain proteins; when not cleared fully by the liver, it accumulates and irritates the arteries.

Fairly recently the medical community came to the realization that inflammation is an underlying cause of or contributor to most chronic diseases, especially coronary artery disease. Years ago, isolated articles in medical journals were the first clues to this. One showed a connection between gum disease and dental decay with heart attacks. Another showed a correlation of heart attacks with the presence of *Helicobacter pylori,* a bacterium that takes shelter in the stomach wall, causing chronic inflammation and sometimes ulcers. Next, diabetes was finally understood as an inflammatory disease, as was smoking. Both were linked to heart attacks. Slowly the dots were connected: inflammation was the link between all the heart-attack risk factors.

Still, doctors thought of inflammation as isolated local phenomena—thus gingivitis, arthritis, and prostatitis are inflammations of the gum, joint, or prostate, respectively—and happened as a response to some insult (trauma, infection, radiation). Today we have a better understanding: the inflammatory system may get turned on in a systemic way, in all your tissues, in your blood, and corrode all your organs. If this happens, whatever system is the weakest point for you will break down first. In the case of heart disease, this is very relevant information. LDL, the so-called "bad cholesterol," could be thought of as the plaster the body uses to repair cracks on the walls of your arteries. When the arteries are cracked, LDL is deposited. This is the beginning of coronary artery disease that may end up in a heart attack or bypass surgery.

Nature has a way of balancing itself out. The way our inflammatory system works is by means of the presence in our blood of both pro-inflammatory factors and anti-inflammatory ones, coexisting in a delicate balance. Inflammation is very necessary when needed so it has to be ready to be sparked into action at the right time. When it is turned on permanently, it is corrosive, so it needs to be turned off immediately when its job is done. The way it is supposed to be balanced is by the foods we eat. Those foods must contain the right balance of pro- and anti-inflammatory nutrients.

Unnatural ways of raising food we consume are only part of the problem. The other part is all the chemicals we add to our foods and our "foodlike" products before they reach the shelves of your local supermarket. When you start considering all the other chemicals that make modern life so apparently "convenient," you start getting the picture and a clue as to why our health is on the decline despite the fact that we have broken the genetic code and invented machines that can show us every millimeter of our anatomy or fix the mechanics of our body when parts collapse. The understanding of toxicity is of paramount importance to the new approach to cardiovascular disease, and it is an issue that will require global change.

Inflammation is the underlying cause that seems to cause cholesterol to be deposited in the arteries and subsequently to break up into clots, followed by heart attacks. Since the Clean program addresses inflammation at its root, cardiovascular disease is the most important beneficiary to this approach of eating less artery-toxic foods, enhanced clearing of homocysteine and uric acid, and correcting the lack of magnesium. Lack of this mineral not only leads to elevated blood pressure, which leads to heart disease, but also makes the nervous system more unstable. Anxiety and stress happen at a lower threshold. This in turn facilitates inflammation, which causes plaque to be deposited in the arteries.

So many of the health problems that eat up money, time, and resources are related to diseases that could be greatly alleviated by looking through detox glasses. My specialty, heart disease, is prime among them: detox programs can help dramatically create the conditions where patients can pave their own paths away from "inevitable" prescription drugs to manage their symptoms.

Of course, there are many scenarios where disease or degeneration has manifested and must be treated with immediate intervention. If the house is burning down, you don't want to waste time collecting papers. You want to put the fire out immediately. It is basic common sense. If you are having a heart attack, you don't want to go to the yoga studio or drink some anti-oxidant tea. You want to get to a hospital immediately and have an angioplasty performed.

EXCEPTIONS TO THE RULE

It is crucially important to treat heart patients with thoughtful care. Many of them are not candidates for a detox (see the contraindications section in "Before You Start Clean" in chapter 7). But sometimes they take matters into their own hands. Who is to say that their instincts are not smarter than my diagnosis? In this spirit I share the "anecdotal" evidence of a patient who used a detox to jump-start his way out of serious cardiovascular disease. Please do not read this as a prediction of any kind of outcome for yourself. It is one man's unique story. But as I always say, anecdotes are worth sharing when it comes to health. They can be windows into the miraculous.

When I was living in Venice, California, I once saw a patient who refused to submit to any tests or take any medications with such conviction that it was impossible for me to persuade him to take anything. And if someone needed Western medicine the day I saw him, it was him. He came to me with classic symptoms of unstable angina. This means, chest pain on and off, very likely caused by an unstable plaque in the coronary artery tree. An unstable plaque is one that ruptures so that blood clots are forming and dissolving, threatening to cause a heart attack. If the clots do not dissolve (our blood is constantly dissolving clots) a heart attack is inevitable. My first recommendation was that he chew and swallow an aspirin to prevent a blood clot from forming and that as he did that, I would call for an ambulance that would take him to the nearest hospital. There, an angiogram and an angioplasty (and most likely a stent) could save his life and bridge things until slower solutions, like right nutrition and exercise, could take effect.

He so adamantly refused even an aspirin that I decided to help him in other ways. I gave him grapeseed extract to thin his blood, fish oils to counteract inflammation and also prevent clotting, and magnesium to stabilize the nerve and electric cells in the heart, which are the cells that form the heart's electrical system, needed to coordinate contraction. I told him to rest and started him on a strict green juice fast.

Statins for Everybody?

It is shocking to read new reports regarding statins. Going one step further than the madness of automatically dispensing statins to everyone with elevated cholesterol without first lowering the levels naturally, now they want to give statins even to people with low cholesterol as a preventive measure, because statins will somehow reduce inflammation. Since one of the main reasons for inflammation is the accumulation of toxins, if the liver is not clearing up toxins at an optimal rate, isn't it much more natural to improve its function than to block it further with statins? One of the side effects of statins is actually to inhibit an important reaction in the liver, making the whole problem worse. Furthermore, statins may just destroy liver cells completely; that's why we need to get blood tests to monitor liver enzymes when taking them.

I called him literally every thirty minutes for the first two days and made him promise me that if the chest pain became permanent or worse, and if he had any other symptom, he would allow me to call an ambulance. It was not necessary. After a day his chest pain went away. After a week he felt so good he started ex-

There is a place for statins in our toolbox. Sometimes the whole thing is so messed up that we need to block a survival mechanism (cholesterol making) that may end up killing us. Yes statins do stabilize arterial plaque and prevent heart attacks, and I use them in these cases. But I try to use them as a bridge, while I guide my patients to make the changes (dietary and exercise) that will later allow them to discontinue the statins. Certainly there are cases in which genetic defects or simply the inability to make those changes warrant the use of statins as a long-term plan, and thank God for them. But in today's world, in the vast majority of cases in which we use statins so freely the patient would be much better served by basic measures, including detoxification and liver function enhancement. For this reason, cleansing and detoxification are very useful tools in my toolbox for my daily cardiology practice.

ercising, against my advice. He juiced for three weeks and then went to raw foods. Four years later he is still on a health kick, has never had chest pain again, and has lost thirty pounds. I will never know exactly what happened but I bet my medical title he reversed his own heart disease.

This story is not to encourage anyone to do a detox program when they have chest pain that suggests coronary artery disease. On the contrary, I still give this patient a piece of my mind when I see him about how he risked his life, and my medical license, on that occasion. But one cannot argue with good results, and he had them. There are rules and there are "exceptions to the rules," and in this moment in time when everything we know about staying healthy is changing, it's possible that more people could be exceptions than they think.

CHAPTER TEN

A Vision of the Future

The future of medicine is NO medicine.
If monkeys one day lost the instincts telling them
to eat bananas, would there suddenly be
monkey nutritionists?

The wide variety of diseases the human species is prey to, the severity of many of them, and the suffering experienced as a consequence by our loved ones, our communities, and the entire race are exclusive to mankind. In nature, most animals are born, roam, eat, reproduce, and die from old age, from injury, or at the jaws of other animals. There is no cancer, heart disease, diabetes, depression and autoimmune diseases affecting wild animals. These things are a human phenomenon. We are paying a high price for extracting ourselves from nature and putting the whole planet at our service. Wildlife is now suffering the consequences as well and we are threatening to make life on the planet disappear.

It will take more than the Clean program and the follow-up maintenance to completely undo and prevent the damaging effects that modern life has on our biology, but at least we as individuals can avoid becoming part of the alarming statistics. We can avoid being one of the projected 20 million annual new cancer cases predicted worldwide by 2030—up from 12 million a year today—and sidestep the degenerative conditions that have made "growing old" into a disease of its own. When I was younger, "cancer" was something that friends of friends had. Today, there are at least ten people in my close circle of friends who are attempting to survive it. This is not a fear tactic to get anybody to complete Clean or any other detoxification program, or even to make any of the changes recommended in this book. It is simply a report of the reality we are living in. It will take a radical planet-wide shift in all areas of human endeavor to bring back the balance of health to a centered place. It demands effort. It is inconvenient. But it is essential to recognize the need for such a shift.

Global warming was the first "inconvenient truth" to hit critical mass awareness. Finally, we are stepping up to the plate to meet its challenges. Global toxicity is another inconvenient truth, and it needs as much attention and as many innovative solutions in action as the first one if we are to survive as a species and flourish. Delivering some of these solutions is my intention with this book and with Clean. To raise awareness, and provide safe and simple tools for you to live a more vibrant life, look broadly for solutions to your health issues, and explore other areas of wellness.

There is no question that the health-care system as it is in the West right now is failing us. To return to the analogy of the earth as a living animal whose lungs are the forests and the Internet its nervous system, then the hospitals are its lymph nodes—the sites where diseases should be stopped and healing should happen. But the lymph nodes are not doing this job; instead of making people better, we have to ask if modern medicine's reliance on expensive drugs, surgery, and expensive intervention might just be making them sicker. It is certainly breeding an atmosphere of distrust and even fear. In my own work as a cardiologist in some extremely busy hospitals, I have frequently met with patients who were terrified about their own impending treatments. They had had friends or family members who had undergone similar surgeries and suffered medical neglect, and gotten "iatrogenic" illnesses (the recently coined term given to sicknesses that come from modern medicine, whether from harmful drug interactions or medical mistakes). Sometimes these people had been affected fatally. The undercurrent of anger and stress in our places of healing today is rarely discussed but it is often felt by doctors.

There is a great need to return the power to patients so they can see that in fact they are in charge of their own well-being and health. A doctor or a hospital team doesn't cure anything; we help create the conditions whereby the body can best heal itself. My own experience of losing digestive health and falling into depression, then fixing the digestion through cleansing and restoring the intestinal tract, and losing the depression as a result, was a revelation. Since that time I have witnessed countless people not only lose weight and troubling symptoms by detoxing but also gain the confidence in their own potential to heal, as I did.

My meditation teacher used to say, by way of encouraging her students to perform service in the school of meditation's kitchen, "First, we comfort the belly, and then we talk spirituality." She meant that when physical health is firmly established, the spirit can then begin to expand and grow. When you commit to your first cleanse, transformation on every level is facilitated. This is reflected by patients, even the most skeptical ones, who tell me their detox program has liberated something beyond physical energy. Often it has revealed a new spaciousness inside. When attention is released from food for a while, other subtler activities, such as contemplating, dreaming, and reflecting, are funded. Many times the simple fact of reducing time spent on meals has recaptured time for other important things such as spending more time with their children, creative projects, or spiritual lives. They say, "I've remembered what's important in my life."

In this respect, Clean can be the beginning of a great awakening. Some years ago I met an Indian saint who was famous for producing glittering bangles from thin air to give to his delighted followers. When asked why he would do that instead of only lecturing on the yogic scriptures, he said, "First I give them what they want with the hope that one day they will want what I really have to give them." Likewise with a detox program, when you come to it to put some shinier, healthier, younger-looking "leaves" on your tree, you cannot help but clean up the roots also. This triggers a positive cascade: it builds a foundation for ongoing good health. This in turn opens the way to gain the peace in body and mind where true happiness is anchored. Ultimately, it is by building this real, enduring health that we will cure the fever of global toxicity affecting us, our planet, and our future.

CHAPTER ELEVEN

The Clean Recipes

21 Liquid Meals: Smoothies, Soups, and Juices

The following recipes make two servings each. You may either make the full recipe, and save half for later (store in fridge and use within 24 hours), or make half the recipe.

SMOOTHIES

If possible, make your ice from pure filtered water. If you prefer your smoothies less chilled, leave out the ice. All fruit may be fresh or frozen. First, here are two recipes, for nut milk and coconut milk, which you can use in the smoothie recipes.

Basic Coconut Milk (makes about 4 cups)

It is simple to make your own supply of coconut milk.

    1 cup of dried, unsweetened coconut

    4 cups of warm pure water

1. Soak the coconut in the water for fifteen minutes.
2. Strain through a fine strainer.

In any recipes that call for coconut milk you may substitute the same amount of coconut water blended with 5 to 6 macadamia nuts or ¼ avocado, for extra body.

Basic Nut Milk (makes 4 cups)

Use this recipe to make the almond milk required in some the following recipes, as well as brazil-nut milk, and many others. Do not use peanuts.

    1 cup of nuts, soaked for 3 hours in purified water

    1 teaspoon vanilla powder or extract

    1 to 2 teaspoons agave syrup or brown rice syrup

    3 cups purified water

1. Drain the nuts, discarding water.
2. Place in blender with vanilla powder or extract, sweetener, and 3 cups purified water.
3. Blend for about 3 minutes.
4. Strain through fine strainer or cheesecloth.

5. Store in refrigerator; lasts for 2 days.

Agave syrup, also called agave nectar, is made from cactus. It is still a sugar (fructose) so use it sparingly.

Green Smoothie

   1½ cups of almond milk (see recipe for Basic Nut Milk)

   ½ cup of coconut water (fresh if possible; see note on coconut water)

   2 leaves lacinato (dark green) kale or Swiss chard, coarsely chopped

   ¼ avocado

   ½ cup mango chunks

   ½ cup of ice

1. Blend together until smooth.

Coconut water is the clear liquid inside a fresh coconut. Fresh coconuts can be bought at health food stores and some supermarkets. If you don't have a coconut, you can buy coconut water in packs in a supermarket; look for the O.N.E. brand.

If using commercial almond milk instead of homemade, try to get a kind that contains no soy. Blue Diamond unsweetened vanilla almond milk is one option.

Kale, Pineapple, and Chia Smoothie

Chia is a superfood seed with complete protein and omega-3 and omega-6 fatty acids. Soaking for a few hours in pure water will activate the enzymes, but is not essential.

When juicing kale, look for the darkest-green kind with long leaves, such as lacinato or dinosaur kale. If it's not available, use any kale you can find.

½ cup pineapple chunks

2 leaves lacinato kale

2 teaspoons soaked chia seeds

1 cup pure water

1 to 2 teaspoons agave syrup

½ cup ice

1. Blend together until smooth.

Mango and Coconut Milk Smoothie

1 cup mango chunks

½ cup pineapple chunks

1½ cups coconut milk

1 to 2 teaspoons agave syrup

½ cup ice

1. Blend together until smooth.

Coconut milk is not the same as coconut water. It is made from pureeing and soaking the white meat of a fresh coconut. Canned versions may have additives; read ingredients and when in doubt make your own.

Blueberry, Carob, and Almond Milk Smoothie

    1 cup blueberries

    1½ cups almond milk (see recipe for Basic Nut
      Milk)

    1 to 2 teaspoons agave syrup

    2 teaspoons raw cacao powder, carob powder, or
      cocoa

    ½ cup ice

1. Blend together until smooth.

Cacao powder is the same thing as cocoa powder, but the raw form is usually called cacao. It is preferable because it's packed with nutrients, including magnesium, and is high in antioxidants. The Navitas Naturals brand is stocked in many health food stores.

Energy Smoothie with Almond Butter and Cardamom

    ¼ cup almond butter

    2 cardamom pods or 1 teaspoon ground cardamom

    1½ cups of pure water

    1 cup frozen peaches

    1 to 2 teaspoons agave syrup

    ½ cup ice

1. Blend together until smooth.

Tahini or pumpkin-seed butter can be substituted for almond butter.

Berry Smoothie with Coconut Milk and Cinnamon

 2 cups mixed blueberries and raspberries
 2 cups coconut milk with coconut meat or ¼
  avocado added
  to 1½ cups coconut milk
 1 teaspoon cinnamon
 1 to 2 teaspoons agave
 ½ cup ice

1. Blend together until smooth.

Dig some white coconut meat out of a fresh coconut, available at natural food stores.

Tropical Smoothie

 1½ cups pineapple and mango chunks
 2 tablespoons passion fruit puree
 1½ cups any kind of nut milk (see recipe for Basic
  Nut Milk)
 ½ cup ice

1. Blend together until smooth.
2. Add 1 sprig of mint if desired.

Look for frozen packs of passion fruit puree or substitute extra pineapple chunks if not available.

SOUPS

Chilled Cucumber Soup with Mint

3 cucumbers, peeled and seeded

1 lemon, peeled

¼ cup pine nuts

4 cups pure water

¼ cup fresh mint leaves

1 teaspoon sea salt

2 tablespoons olive oil

1. Blend everything except fresh mint together in a high-speed blender for 3 minutes or until smooth.
2. Add mint and blend for 15 seconds.
3. Serve chilled.

Use sun-dried sea salt or pink Himalayan salt if possible.

Spinach and Dulse Soup

1 zucchini, cut in ½ cubes

1 stalk celery

1 scallion

1 tablespoon extra virgin olive oil

¼ cup dulse flakes

¼ avocado

2 cups spinach leaves, washed

4 cups pure water

1. Blend together in a high-speed blender for 3 minutes or until smooth.
2. Season with sea salt to taste.
3. Serve with garnish of dulse and a drizzle of olive oil.

Dulse is a sea vegetable; look for it in the ethnic foods aisle of your supermarket or in a health food store.

Easy Pineapple and Avocado Gazpacho

2 cups pineapple, diced small

1 avocado, diced small

½ to 1 jalapeño chili pepper, seeds removed and chopped fine

½ teaspoon sea salt

Juice of 1 lime

Sprouts or cilantro (garnish)

1. Combine all ingredients except garnish in a bowl.
2. Put half of the mixture in the blender and blend.
3. Pour blended mixture into the bowl and fold in to unblended diced avocado and pineapple.

4. Add ½ cup water if thinner texture is desired.

5. Serve chilled garnished with sprouts or cilantro.

Sprouts are a living food, rich in enzymes. Look for them in the produce section of your supermarket. Sunflower sprouts are especially good, if you can find them.

Zucchini and Basil Soup

1 zucchini, diced

1 stalk celery

1 tablespoon red or sweet onion, finely chopped

1 tablespoon extra virgin olive oil

5 basil leaves

½ teaspoon sea salt

¼ avocado

4 cups pure water

Additional basil leaves (for garnish)

1. Blend all together in a high-speed blender.

2. Garnish with fresh basil leaves, finely shredded.

Butternut Squash Bisque

1½ cups butternut squash, peeled and diced

2 stalks celery, diced

1 tablespoon red or sweet onion, chopped

½ cup yellow zucchini or crookneck squash
  (summer squash), diced

1 tablespoon extra virgin olive oil

1 teaspoon sea salt

¼ teaspoon turmeric

1 teaspoon of apple cider vinegar

4 cups water

Fresh parsley, sprouts, or sunflower seeds (garnish)

1. Blend all together except garnish.
2. Check seasoning.
3. Serve and garnish with fresh parsley or sprouts and sunflower seeds.
4. Fresh chilis may be added for added spice if desired.

Apple and Butternut Squash Soup

2 cups butternut squash, peeled and chopped

2 stalks celery

2 green apples, peeled

¼ cup pine nuts

1 teaspoon apple cider vinegar

½ teaspoon sea salt

¼ cup fresh tarragon, chopped

4 to 5 cups pure water

1. Blend all ingredients except tarragon in a high-speed blender.
2. Check seasoning.

3. Add the tarragon and blend again for 10 seconds, just enough for it to be mixed in.
4. Serve in a bowl or mug slightly warm or at room temperature.

Carrot and Ginger Soup

1½ cups butternut squash, peeled and diced
2 cups diced carrots
1½ cups diced yellow squash
¼ cup chopped red onion
¼ cup sliced celery
2 tablespoons extra virgin olive oil
1½ tablespoons apple cider vinegar
1 teaspoon sea salt
Juice of 2-inch piece of ginger, passed through a juicer
4 cups pure water
Additional olive oil and chopped herbs (garnish)

1. Blend all together in a high-speed blender for about 3 minutes, or until smooth.
2. Serve either slightly warm or at room temperature.
3. Drizzle with a little olive oil and freshly chopped herbs.

JUICES

Pass the fruits and vegetable combinations given through a juicer. All of these juices can be served immediately or stored in the fridge in a glass jar with a lid. Use within one day.

Green Juice

2 green apples

3 stalks celery

1 leaf lacinato kale

1 leaf Swiss chard

¼ cabbage

1 head broccoli

½ medium cucumber

½ lemon

Apple, Kale, Sunflower Sprout, and Radish Juice

2 apples

2 cups of sunflower or other sprouts

½ medium cucumber

1 leaf kale

1 cup daikon white radish or red radish slices

1 lemon, peeled (optional; for extra taste)

Apple, Ginger, Lemon, and Spinach Juice

2 green apples

½-inch piece of fresh ginger

1 lemon, peeled

1 cup spinach leaves

Carrot, Beet, Cabbage, and Watercress Juice

2 medium carrots

¼ white cabbage

1 small beet

1 cup watercress leaves

Fennel and Apple Juice

2 green apples

2 heads of fennel

½ lemon, peeled

Cucumber, Cabbage, and Parsley Juice

1 medium cucumber, peeled if not organic

2 cups shredded white cabbage

1 cup parsley

½ lemon, peeled

Pineapple, Lime, and Fresh Mint Juice

2 to 3 cups pineapple chunks

1 lime, peeled

¼ cup fresh mint

21 Solid Meals

All these recipes are for two servings. If you are cooking for yourself and a partner who is not doing Clean, he or she will enjoy the food and can add desired side dishes. If you are cooking for yourself, you can keep one portion for the next day, or halve the recipe.

Use organic, hormone-free chicken and lamb and wild-caught fish if possible. Avoid farmed fish.

Unless otherwise noted, you can serve some raw, steamed, or sautéed greens (kale, spinach, chard) as side dishes to these meals, or other vegetables allowed on the Elimination Diet.

MEALS WITH FISH

Watercress and Shaved Fennel Salad with Seared Tuna

2 (4-ounce) pieces of fresh tuna, ½-inch thick, or
  1 can tuna in water
2 cups fresh watercress, washed
½ cup avocado, diced medium
1 bulb fennel, shaved thinly
1 cup green beans, sliced
2 tablespoons olive oil

3 to 4 black olives per person

Juice of 1 lemon

1 teaspoon sea salt

1. Combine all ingredients except tuna in a bowl and toss.
2. If using fresh fish, heat the grill to high. A sauté pan will work also.
3. Brush fish with olive oil and season.
4. Sear for 2 minutes on each side.
5. Serve salad in a mound on flat plates with tuna sliced or flaked on top.

Steamed Bass with Fennel, Parsley, and Capers

2 (5-ounce) portions of striped bass

1 fennel bulb, sliced thinly

¼ cup Italian parsley, chopped

1 tablespoon capers, rinsed

½ lemon, juiced

½ teaspoon sea salt

¼ medium white onion, sliced

2 tablespoons extra virgin olive oil

Additional olive oil and chopped fresh parsley (garnish)

1. Put onion, fennel, and lemon juice in a medium saucepan and cover with one inch of water.

2. Bring to boil and simmer for 5 minutes.
3. Remove from heat and put in the 2 portions of fish, seasoned with sea salt.
4. Sprinkle with capers and parsley and cover the pan.
5. Simmer for about 8 to 10 minutes, until fish is almost flaky.
6. Place the vegetables in the bottom of a shallow bowl and the fish on top, drizzle with olive oil and sprinkle with fresh parsley. Serve one cup of steamed brown rice per person on the side, if desired.

Roast Salmon with Broccoli Rabe and Quinoa

2 (5-ounce) portions of wild salmon, seasoned with ½ teaspoon sea salt
1 bunch of broccoli rabe, washed, stalks trimmed and split lengthwise
2 cloves garlic, sliced lengthwise
2 tablespoons extra virgin olive oil
1 cup cooked quinoa

1. Heat oven to 400°F.
2. Heat a skillet and add 1 tablespoon of the olive oil.
3. When oil is hot, add salmon and sear on one side for 3 minutes. Flip over, sear other side for 1 more minute, then remove from pan.

4. Place on baking tray and place in oven for 7 to 8 minutes.
5. Drain excess oil from skillet, heat skillet again, and add the remainder of the olive oil.
6. Sauté the garlic for 1 minute.
7. Turn heat down to medium. Place broccoli rabe in pan, add ¼ cup water, cover, and steam for 2 minutes.
8. Serve the greens on a platter with the salmon on top. Serve quinoa as a side dish.

Halibut Baked in Parchment with Olives and Thyme

2 (5-ounce) portions of halibut
¼ cup of pitted, halved kalamata olives
2 sprigs of thyme
1 lemon, sliced thinly in discs, skin on
1 zucchini, sliced thin diagonally
2 tablespoons extra virgin olive oil
Sea salt
Parchment paper cut into two 12-inch circles

1. Heat oven to 425°F.
2. Brush each parchment sheet with oil.
3. Place one piece of halibut in the middle of each sheet.

4. Season with sea salt.
5. On top of the fish place three thin slices of lemon and three slices of zucchini between the slices of lemon, then top with a sprig of thyme.
6. Sprinkle the olives over the top and drizzle with olive oil.
7. Pull the sides of the parchment together like a calzone. Fold paper over and crinkle together to seal.
8. Place each package on a baking tray and place in the lower third of the oven.
9. Bake for 12 to 15 minutes; the paper will puff up and brown lightly.
10. Remove from oven and place on plates to serve. Open packages at the table.

If you have no parchment paper, use a covered oven-proof dish.

Warm Salmon and Asparagus Salad with Pesto

2 (5-ounce) portions of wild salmon
2 tablespoons fresh pesto
1 bunch asparagus, woody ends trimmed off
4 cups mesclun greens or arugula
Extra virgin olive oil
Lemon

For the pesto:

2 bunches fresh basil, washed and leaves pulled from the hard stalks

¼ cup pine nuts

½ cup extra virgin olive oil

1 clove garlic

Sea salt for seasoning

1. To make the pesto, place basil, pine nuts, and garlic in a food processor and process on medium.
2. Drizzle in the olive oil while the motor is running.
3. Season with salt.
4. If it is too thick, add a small amount of pure water (¼ cup at most).
5. Set aside in a bowl.
6. Turn grill on high. If you don't have a grill, use your oven's broiler.
7. Brush each piece of salmon with olive oil and season with salt and pepper.
8. Do the same with the asparagus.
9. Grill the asparagus first, for 2 minutes on each side. Set aside.
10. Grill the salmon for 3 minutes on each side.
11. Prepare the salad. Place the greens in a bowl, toss with olive oil, salt, and lemon juice.
12. Place on two plates.

13. Arrange the asparagus nicely on one side and the salmon on the other.

14. Drizzle 1 tablespoon of pesto over the top of each piece of salmon.

15. Serve while the salmon is still warm.

You may used prepared pesto as long as it doesn't contain any additives.

Asian-Flavored Tuna with Stir-Fried Vegetables

10 ounces tuna or yellowtail, cut into 1-inch chunks

½ cup nama shoyu or wheat-free tamari (gluten-free soy sauce)

2 cloves garlic, crushed

2 teaspoons maple syrup

1-inch piece of fresh ginger, sliced thinly

1 carrot, sliced on the diagonal

1 baby bok choy, sliced lengthwise

1 cup broccoli, cut small

1 zucchini, sliced on the diagonal

1 teaspoon sesame oil

1 tablespoon olive oil

1. Mix tamari or nama shoyu, ginger, garlic, and maple syrup in a bowl.

2. Put tuna chunks in it; let marinate for a few minutes.

3. Divide chunks evenly and thread onto 2 skewers.

4. Turn broiler to high. When it is heated up, place skewers under it and cook for 1 to 2 minutes.

5. Turn and cook for 1 to 2 more minutes, then set aside.

6. Heat a sauté pan on high heat.

7. Add the olive and sesame oils.

8. Add all the vegetables except the bok choy.

9. Use a wooden spoon to help coat the vegetables with oil and stir them for 2 minutes as they cook.

10. Add the bok choy and ¼ cup water.

11. Cover for 1 minute, allow vegetables to steam slightly.

12. Place vegetables in a flat bowl and top with tuna skewers.

You can also replace the tuna with a white fish such as striped bass or cod.

Note: Small amounts of fermented soy such as tamari are good for the digestion, so very limited use such as in these recipes is fine, even though you are eliminating soy in general during Clean.

Snapper Cooked with Capers, Lemon, and Fresh Thyme, Served with Swiss Chard

2 (6-ounce) filets of snapper, pin bones removed

¼ cup capers

Grated zest from one lemon

2 sprigs of thyme

1 tablespoon extra virgin olive oil

Sea salt

4 cups of Swiss chard, washed and roughly chopped

1. Heat the oven to 425°F.
2. In a baking dish, place the snapper, grated lemon zest, capers, and thyme.
3. Drizzle olive oil over the top.
4. Season with salt and pepper.
5. Cover with foil.
6. Bake for 15 minutes, then remove from oven.
7. Heat a sauté pan and add 1 tablespoon olive oil.
8. When hot, add the Swiss chard; cover and let steam for 2 minutes.
9. Serve the fish on a bed of chard.
10. Spoon juices and capers over the fish. Garnish with a sprig of fresh thyme.

You can substitute a local white fish.

MEALS WITH CHICKEN OR LAMB

Roast Chicken with Balsamic Vinegar, Garlic, and Rosemary Wild Rice Pilaf

Cook chicken breasts with skin on for flavor, then remove skin before eating.

2 chicken breasts

2 cloves garlic, sliced thinly lengthwise

1½ cups balsamic vinegar

2 tablespoons minced rosemary

2 tablespoons extra virgin olive oil

1 teaspoon sea salt

2 cups cooked wild rice, made with a vegetable stock

2 scallions, thinly sliced

¼ cup cilantro, chopped

¼ cup fresh mint, chopped

¼ cup sunflower seeds, soaked for 2 hours

1. Heat oven to 425°F.
2. In a small saucepan reduce the balsamic vinegar by simmering and stirring occasionally until it becomes the consistency of a syrup.
3. Add the garlic and rosemary and simmer for 2 minutes more. Set aside.
4. Brush the chicken breasts with olive oil and salt.

5. Place on a baking tray and roast in oven for 10 minutes.

6. Brush with generous amounts of balsamic mixture.

7. Turn the oven down to 375°F and roast for a further 10 minutes.

8. Brush again with balsamic mixture and cook 2 minutes more.

9. Remove from oven and let cool slightly, remove the skins and thinly slice.

10. To make the pilaf, place chicken, rice, scallions, cilantro, mint, and sunflower seeds in a bowl.

11. Mix together and season with salt and pepper.

Depending on the season, you may want to serve this at room temperature or warm. Soaking sunflower seeds activates the enzymes, making the seeds easier to digest.

Stir-Fried Vegetables and Chicken with Buckwheat Noodles

    1 packet of buckwheat noodles (to make about
      2 cups when cooked)
    1 teaspoon salt
    1 teaspoon sesame oil
    2 carrots, sliced thinly on an angle
    1 cup broccoli florets

1 cup snap peas

1 cup baby bok choy, sliced lengthwise

1 cup sliced zucchini cut on an angle

3 scallions, sliced into 2-inch pieces on the bias

2 cloves garlic

¼ cup sliced ginger

1 tablespoon nama shoyu or wheat-free tamari

2 chicken breasts, grilled and sliced

1. In a large pot boil 6 cups of water; add the salt.
2. Add the noodles, reduce heat slightly, and boil for about 3 minutes or until tender.
3. Place noodles in a colander and rinse thoroughly in cold water.
4. Drain water completely, toss lightly in the sesame oil, and set aside.
5. For the stir-fry, heat a heavy skillet and add olive oil.
6. Keep on a high heat and add garlic and ginger for one minute, stir with a wooden spoon.
7. Add the rest of the vegetables a little at a time to keep heat up, except the snap peas.
8. Toss, flip or just use a wooden spoon to coat vegetables and prevent scorching.
9. Add the nama shoyu and 2 tablespoons water.
10. Finally, add the snap peas for 1 minute.

11. Toss in a bowl with the noodles and serve.
12. Garnish with fresh cilantro. Serve chicken breasts on the side.

Quinoa Salad with Chicken and Mixed Greens

2 cups cooked and cooled quinoa

2 (4-ounce) chicken breasts, grilled or steamed and thinly sliced

1 tablespoon chopped parsley

¼ cup currants

¼ cup chopped raw almonds

½ cup diced carrots

¼ cup chopped mint

¼ cup scallions, cut thinly diagonally

¼ cup chopped parsley

¼ cup lime

1 teaspoon agave nectar

½ teaspoon ground cumin

1 teaspoon sea salt

½ cup olive oil

4 cups salad greens tossed with 2 tablespoons olive oil

1. Steam chicken breast: cook it in ½-inch boiling water in a covered pan for 6 minutes.

2. Put all ingredients except chicken and salad greens in a bowl, and toss together with quinoa, adjust seasoning to taste.

3. Mound half this quinoa salad on each plate.

4. Make a bed of salad greens next to quinoa and place the sliced chicken on top.

Roasted Lamb Chops with Rosemary and Steamed Asparagus

½ pound asparagus

½ teaspoon salt

4 lamb chops or 1 rack of lamb (about 7 chops)

Fresh rosemary, finely chopped

2 cloves garlic, finely chopped

1 tablespoon extra virgin olive oil

Salt and ground pepper

1 tablespoon Dijon mustard

1. Trim the woody ends off the asparagus. You may also peel off about 1 inch of the tough green fibrous sheath from the base of the asparagus stalks with a vegetable peeler.

2. Put 1 inch of water and ½ teaspoon sea salt in a saucepan and bring to a boil. Place asparagus in the pan and steam for about 3 minutes, until tender but not soft (al dente). Drain and set aside.

4. Make a paste of the olive oil, rosemary, garlic, and Dijon mustard.

5. Brush the lamb chops with the paste.

6. Using high heat, grill, sauté, or broil the lamb chops for 3 to 4 minutes on each side for medium-rare.

7. Remove from heat and allow to rest.

8. Place asparagus on a plate and arrange the lamb chops.

For a delicious additional flavor note, roast some garlic cloves in a small oven-proof dish at 350°F for 30 minutes and serve with lamb chops.

Grilled Chicken Breast with Grilled Vegetables

2 (4-ounce) skinless chicken breasts

3 tablespoons olive oil

1 zucchini cut diagonally into about 6 pieces

1 yellow squash cut diagonally into about 6 pieces

1 portobello mushroom, cut in half

1 teaspoon nama shoyu or wheat-free tamari

6 asparagus spears trimmed and sliced

4 scallions

1. Combine nama shoyu or tamari and 1 tablespoon of the olive oil and marinate mushroom in mixture.

2. Heat the grill or broiler to high. Brush the chicken with 1 tablespoon olive oil and season lightly.

3. Place all the vegetables except mushroom halves in a bowl and toss with 1 tablespoon olive oil, salt, and pepper.

4. Grill the vegetables about 1½ minutes each side and set aside.

5. Grill the portobello mushroom pieces for 2 minutes on both sides.

6. Grill the chicken breasts for about 3 minutes on each side.

7. Make a bed of the grilled vegetables and place the chicken on top.

Parsley- and Mustard-Flavored Lamb Loin and Spinach Salad

2 pieces of trimmed lamb loin, about 4 ounces each

¼ cup Dijon mustard

1 clove garlic, minced

1 cup parsley, chopped fine

Sea salt and black pepper, to taste

4 cups of baby organic spinach

¼ cup black Mediterranean olives

2 tablespoons olive oil

1 tablespoon lemon juice

1. Heat the oven to 425°F.
2. Make a paste of garlic, Dijon mustard, and parsley.
3. Generously cover the lamb with the paste and season with salt and pepper. Let sit for half an hour on a baking tray to let meat absorb flavor.
4. Place in oven, uncovered, for about 15 minutes. Turn the meat.
5. Cook for another 5 minutes. Meat should be medium done.
6. Let rest for 5 minutes, then slice into about ⅛-inch slices with a sharp knife.
7. Prepare the salad. In a bowl, toss the spinach with the olive oil and lemon.
8. Place salad on 2 plates and add the olives.
9. Arrange the lamb slices over the spinach and serve.

Moroccan Spiced Lamb Served with Quinoa and Wilted Greens

¼ teaspoon ground cumin
¼ teaspoon ground cardamom
¼ teaspoon freshly ground pepper
¼ teaspoon ground ginger
Pinch cayenne pepper
¼ teaspoon cinnamon
1½ teaspoons sea salt
2 garlic cloves, minced

4 lamb rib chops

2 tablespoons olive oil

1 tablespoon chopped parsley and mint

4 cups steamed mustard greens or kale

2 cups cooked quinoa

1. In a small bowl mix the spices with the sea salt.
2. Pat the garlic all over the lamb chops, then sprinkle them with the spice mixture.
3. In a large skillet, heat the vegetable oil. Add the chops and cook over moderately high heat, turning once, for about 6 minutes for medium-rare.
4. Transfer the chops to two plates, garnish with the parsley and mint. Serve the quinoa on the side.

VEGETARIAN MEALS

Macro Bowl with Rice or Quinoa and Ginger-Miso Dressing

2 (2-inch) wedges of kabucha squash, seeds removed

1 cup of cauliflower florets

2 baby bok choys, cut into 4 lengthwise, or 2 cups other greens (kale, collards, Swiss chard)

2 cups cooked quinoa or brown rice

2 cups of cooked or canned salt- and additive-free
adzuki beans

1 cup soaked hijiki or wakame seaweed

Fresh cilantro leaves (for garnish)

1-inch piece of ginger

1 clove garlic

¼ cup white sweet miso

Juice of 1 lemon

¼ cup olive oil

1 teaspoon of agave if a sweeter taste is desired

1. Place the kabucha squash in a steamer or saucepan
   with a steaming rack set over boiling water; steam
   for 3 minutes.
2. Arrange the remaining vegetables, so you can
   assemble bowl nicely, in the steamer for about 3
   minutes.
3. In individual serving bowls, arrange the beans,
   the rice or quinoa, the greens, and squash pieces
   pointing in four directions.
4. On top place the hijiki or wakame. Garnish with
   sprouts or fresh cilantro leaves just for color.
5. To make the ginger-miso dressing, in a food
   processor blend ginger, garlic, miso, lemon juice,
   olive oil, and agave, if used. If desired, add a little
   water for a thinner consistency.

6. Serve the dressing on the side.

Hijiki and wakame seaweed can be found in your supermarket's Asian section or in an Asian market or a health food store.

Tri-Salad Platter of Hummus, Tabbouleh, and Marinated Kale

Heap half of each of the following salads on a plate and serve with cucumber and carrot slices

Hummus
1 cup cooked chick peas, drained
¼ cup tahini
Juice of 1 lemon
¼ teaspoon salt
¼ teaspoon ground cumin
1 clove garlic
2 tablespoons olive oil
Sea salt to taste
Paprika to garnish

1. Place all ingredients in a food processor and process for 2 minutes. Add ¼ cup or more water if necessary. Season. Place in bowl and sprinkle paprika on top.

Quinoa Tabbouleh

2 cups cooked quinoa

1 tablespoon chopped parsley

¼ cup currants

¼ cup chopped raw almonds

½ cup diced carrots

¼ cup chopped mint

¼ cup scallions diagonally cut thinly

¼ cup chopped parsley

¼ cup lime juice

1 teaspoon agave nectar

½ teaspoon ground cumin

1 teaspoon sea salt

½ cup olive oil

1. Mix all ingredients in a bowl and let sit for 20 minutes before serving to allow flavors to blend.

Marinated Kale with Radish and Pine Nuts

2 cups shredded lacinato (dark-green) kale, ribs removed

4 radishes, quartered

2 tablespoons pine nuts

Olive oil

Juice of ½ lemon

Sea salt

1. In a bowl combine all ingredients and marinate.

Lentil Salad

- 1 cup dried green lentils
- ½ teaspoon cumin
- ¼ teaspoon turmeric
- 1 tablespoon ginger, freshly grated
- 1 clove garlic, crushed
- Juice of 1 lime
- ¼ cup pineapple, diced small
- ¼ cup olive oil
- ½ teaspoon sea salt
- 1 cup zucchini, diced
- 1 cup cucumber, diced
- ¾ cup carrots, diced
- ¼ cup cilantro leaves, pulled off stems and chopped
- ¼ cup scallions
- 2 cups salad greens, washed and dried

1. Place dried lentils in 3 cups water and simmer, covered, for 30 minutes.
2. When tender, remove from heat and drain.
3. Set aside to cool.
4. To make the dressing, place cumin, turmeric, ginger, garlic, lime juice, olive oil, and sea salt in a glass jar with lid and shake vigorously. Or place all ingredients except pineapple in a food processor

and process until smooth. Add pineapple last so the dressing is chunky.

5. To assemble the salad, place the lentils and all the vegetables, except the greens, in a bowl.

6. Add dressing, mix well, and let sit for 5 minutes to allow the flavors to blend.

7. Serve on top of the greens.

Big Green Salad

½ head romaine lettuce, leaves washed, dried, and torn into
  bite-size pieces

1 bunch of arugula, washed and dried

Dandelion leaves, washed and dried

1 carrot, shredded

6 radishes, cut into 4 pieces each

1 cucumber, cut into 4 pieces lengthwise, then cut into ½-inch chunks

1 avocado, cut into slices

Handful of sunflower sprouts

3 scallions, sliced thin

¼ cup soaked almonds, chopped

1 clove garlic, crushed

Juice of ½ lemon

1 tablespoon apple cider vinegar

1 tablespoon agave syrup

Fresh thyme, basil, and parsley, chopped fine
½ cup grape-seed oil
Salt and pepper

1. To make the dressing, put the lemon juice, garlic, agave syrup, herbs, and grape-seed oil into a glass jar with screw-top lid and shake vigorously.

Season with salt and freshly ground pepper.

2. In a large bowl toss the greens, carrots, radishes, scallions, and cucumber with the dressing.

(You can use individual plates if you choose.)

3. Decorate with the avocado, sprouts, and almonds.

If desired, you may add 2 ounces of shrimp or chicken per portion.

Soaked almonds are easier to digest. To soak almonds, cover in pure water and leave for at least two hours or overnight.

Thai Vegetable Salad Wraps with Almond Sauce

1 tablespoon almond butter
1 teaspoon grated fresh ginger
½ lemon juiced
1 teaspoon of apple cider vinegar
1 clove garlic
1 teaspoon nama shoyu or wheat-free tamari
Pinch of cayenne

⅓ cup pure water

Nori sheets cut into strips ⅛-inch thick by 2
  inches wide

4 large romaine lettuce leaves

½ shredded Napa cabbage

1 carrot, shredded

2 scallions, thinly sliced

6 snow peas, thinly sliced

1 cucumber, peeled, seeded, and thinly sliced

1. To make almond sauce, blend together almond
   butter, ginger, lemon juice, apple cider vinegar,
   garlic, and nama shoyu or tamari until creamy. Add
   more water if too thick.
2. Wash lettuce leaves and set aside to drain.
3. Combine remaining ingredients except nori in a
   bowl.
4. Into each romaine leaf put about one-quarter of
   the mixture and roll up.
5. Drizzle with 1 tablespoon Spicy Almond Sauce per
   wrap.
6. Garnish with cilantro leaf and strips of nori or
   thinly sliced almonds.
7. Serve on a platter.

Adzuki Beans and Brown Rice

1 cup dry adzuki beans, soaked for 2 hours (or use
  additive-free canned beans)

¼ red onion, diced

1 cup diced carrots

½ cup diced celery

1 cup diced butternut or kabucha squash

1 leaf kombu, rinsed well

1 tablespoon extra virgin olive oil

1 cup brown rice, soaked

1½ cups cold water

1. Heat olive oil in a medium-size pot.
2. Sauté the onions, celery, and carrots.
3. Add adzuki beans and kombu and 3 cups water.
4. Bring to boil, reduce heat, and simmer for about 40
   minutes or until beans are tender.
5. Set aside to cool.
6. Place the rice in a pot.
7. Cover and simmer until the water is absorbed,
   about 30 minutes (check on it periodically).
8. Place a scoop of rice in the middle of a bowl.
   Ladle the adzuki beans over it.
9. Garnish with fresh herbs.

The kombu seaweed adds minerals and nutrients; you
can also use wakame.

Vegetarian Nori Rolls with Nut "Rice"

1 cup soaked sunflower seeds

1 cup walnuts, soaked in pure water for 2 hours

¼ red onion

Chopped fresh herbs

1 packet of nori wraps

1 carrot, cut into very thin strips

1 cucumber, peeled, seeded, and cut into thin
  strips

½ avocado, cut into strips

¼ red cabbage, finely shredded

Sprouts

Wheat-free tamari

Wasabi

Fresh ginger

1 tablespoon apple cider vinegar

1 tablespoon water

1. To make the "rice," place the sunflower seeds,
   walnuts, onion, and herbs in a food processor.
   Process for 2 minutes, or until nut mixture has the
   consistency of rice. Set aside.

2. Thinly slice the ginger and marinate in vinegar and
   water.

3. Take a sheet of nori and spread one-fourth of the
   rice mixture onto it.

4. Lay carrot, cucumber, red cabbage, avocado, and sprouts over it.
5. Roll the nori up tightly, using a sushi mat if you have one.
6. Cut the roll into about six pieces, using a sharp knife.
7. Repeat for three more nori sheets.
8. Serve rolls on a platter with marinated ginger, wasabi, and wheat-free tamari

Appendix

Unexpected Common Sources of Heavy-Metal Exposure

ALUMINUM

Aluminum cooking utensils
Baking powder
Antacids (certain brands, see labels)
Antiperspirants
Aluminum cans
Drinking water (alum., used as bactericide)
Milk and milk products (from equipment)
Pickled foods (see labels)
Nasal spray
Toothpaste
Ceramics (AL 203 clay)
Dental amalgams
Cigarette filters, tobacco smoke
Automotive exhausts
Pesticides
Color additives
Vanilla Powder
Table salt, seasonings
Bleached Flour
American cheese
Certain medications
Sutures with wound healing coatings
Rat poison

CADMIUM

Drinking water
Soft water (from galvanized pipes)
Soft drinks
Refined wheat flour
Canned evaporated milk
Processed foods
Oysters
Cigarette smoke, tobacco products
Superphosphate fertilizers
Dental appliances
Ceramic glazes
Paint pigments
Electroplating
Silver polish
Polyvinyl plastics
Rubber carpet backing
Nickel-cadmium batteries
Rust-proofing materials

LEAD

Automobile exhausts (not as much since Pb-free fuels)
Leaded house paints
Drinking water from lead plumbing
Vegetables from Pb-contaminated soil
Canned fruits and juices
Canned evaporated milk

Milk from animals
  fed in Pb-
  contaminated
  land
Bone meal
Organ meats (live)
Lead-arsenic
  pesticides
Leaded caps on
  wine bottles
Rainwater and
  snow
Pottery
Painted glassware
Pencils
Toothpaste
Newsprint
Colored printed
  materials
Eating utensils
Curtain weights
Putty
Car batteries
Firing ranges

MERCURY

Dental amalgams
Broken ther-
  mometers and
  barometers
Grain seeds treated
  with methyl mer-
  cury fungicide
Predator fish, cer-
  tain lake fish
Mercuric chloride
Body powders, talc,
  laxatives
Cosmetics
Latex and solvent-
  thinned paints
Hemorrhoid
  suppositories
Mercurochrome,
  merthiolate
Fabric softeners
Floor waxes and
  polishers
Air conditioner
  filters
Wood preservatives
Certain batteries
Fungicides for lawn
  and shrubs

Leather tanning
  products
Felt
Adhesives
Skin lightening
  creams
Psoriasis ointments
Tattooing
Sewage sludge
  used as fertilizer

ARSENIC

Rat poisons
Insecticide resi-
  dues on fruits and
  vegetables
Drinking wa-
  ter, well water,
  seawater
Automobile
  exhaust
Wine
Household
  detergents
Colored chalk
Sewage disposal
Wood preservatives
Wallpaper dye and
  plaster

Prescription Drugs and Nutritional Depletion

DRUG	NUTRIENT DEPLETIONS	POTENTIAL HEALTH PROBLEMS
ACE inhibitors Captopril (Capoten, Duraclon)	Zinc	Loss of sense of smell and taste, lower immunity, slow wound healing
Beta blockers Propranolol, Metoprolol, Atenolol, Pindolol, Acetutulol Betaxolol, Bisoprolol, Carteolol, Carvedilol, Esmolol, Labetalol, Nadolol, Sotalol, Timolol	Coenzyme Q10 Vitamin B	Congestive heart failure, high blood pressure, low energy Asthma, cardiovascular problems, cramps, osteoporosis, PMS
Cardiac glycosides Digoxin (Lanoxin)	Magnesium Calcium	Depression, edema, irritability, memory loss, muscle weakness Heart/blood pressure irregularities, osteoporosis
Loop diuretics Furosemide (Lasix), Bumetanide (Bumex) Ethacrynic Acid (Edecrin)	Magnesium Potassium Vitamin B1 Vitamin B6	Asthma, cardiovascular problems, cramps Edema, fatigue, irregular heartbeat, muscle weakness Depression, edema, irritability, memory loss, muscle weakness Depression, increased cardiovascular disease risk, sleep disturbance

DRUG	NUTRIENT DEPLETIONS	POTENTIAL HEALTH PROBLEMS
Loop diuretics (continued)	Zinc	Loss of sense of smell and taste, lower immunity, slow wound healing
"Statin" drugs Altorvastatin, Cerivastatin, Lovastatin, Fluvastatin, Pravastatin, Simvastatin	Coenzyme Q10 Beta-carotene	Congestive heart failure, high blood pressure, low energy Vision problems, weakened immunity
	Calcium	Blood clotting, cell wall permeability, enzyme dysfunction, high blood pressure, osteoporosis, rickets
	Folic acid	Anemia, birth defects, cervical dysplasia, elevated homocysteine
	Iron	Hair loss
Cholestyramine	Magnesium	Increased incidence of artheroderosis, heart attacks, hypertension, stroke
	Vitamin A	Vision problems
	Vitamin B12	Anemia, appetite loss, depression, dermatitis, fatigue, nausea, poor blood clotting
	Vitamin D	Hearing loss, muscle weakness, phosphorous retention in kidneys, rheumatic pains
	Vitamin E	Cataracts, dry skin, dry hair, easy bruising, eczema, poor wound healing, PMS

➤

Prescription Drugs and Nutritional Depletion
(continued)

DRUG	NUTRIENT DEPLETIONS	POTENTIAL HEALTH PROBLEMS
Cholestyramine (continued)	Vitamin K	Easy bleeding, rickets and other skeletal disorders
	Zinc	Acne, anorexia, decreased immunity, depression, delayed wound healing, frequent infections, impaired sense of smell and taste
Colestipol	Beta-carotene, Folic acid, Iron, Vitamin A, Vitamin B12, Vitamin D, Vitamin E	See above
Cortiocosteroids Sulfasalazine	Folic acid	Anemia, birth defects, cardiovascular disease, cervical dysplasia
Betamethasone, Budesonide	Calcium	Heart/blood pressure irregularities, tooth decay, osteoporosis
Cortisone, Dexamethasone	Folic acid	Anemia, birth defects, cardiovascular disease, cervical dysplasia
Flunisolide, Fluticasone, Hydrocortisone	Magnesium	Asthma, cardiovascular problems, cramps, PMS
Mometasone, Methylprednisolone	Potassium	Edema, fatigue, irregular heartbeat, muscle weakness

DRUG	NUTRIENT DEPLETIONS	POTENTIAL HEALTH PROBLEMS
Prednison, Prednisolone	Selenium	Lower immunity, reduced antioxidant protection
Triamcinolone	Vitamin C	Easy bruising, lower immunity, poor wound healing
	Vitamin D	Hearing loss, muscle weakness, osteoporosis
	Zinc	Loss of sense of taste and smell, slow wound healing
	Folic acid	Anemia, birth defects, cardiovascular disease, cervical dysplasia
	Magnesium	Asthma, cardiovascular problems, cramps, osteoporosis, PMS
Oral contraceptives	Vitamin B2	Eyes, mucous membranes, nerves, skin problems
	Vitamin B6	Depression, increased cardiovascular disease risk, sleep disturbances
	Vitamin B12	Anemia, increased cardiovascular disease risk, tiredness, weakness
	Vitamin C	Easy bruising, lowered immunity, poor wound healing
	Zinc	Loss of sense of smell and taste, lower immunity, slow wound healing

➤

Prescription Drugs and Nutritional Depletion
(continued)

DRUG	NUTRIENT DEPLETIONS	POTENTIAL HEALTH PROBLEMS
H-2 receptor antagonists Axid, Pepcid, Tagamet, Tritec and Zantac	Calcium	Heart/blood pressure irregularities, osteoporosis, tooth decay
	Folic acid	Anemia, birth defects, cardiovascular disease, cervical dysplasia
	Iron	Anemia, brittle nails, fatigue, hair loss, weakness
	Vitamin B12	Anemia, increased cardio-vascular disease risk, tiredness, weakness
	Vitamin D	Hearing loss, muscle weak ness, osteoporosis
	Zinc	Loss of sense of smell and taste, lowered immunity, slow wound healing
General antibiotics Penicillins, cephalosporins, fluoroquinolones, macrolides, aminoglycosides, sulfonamides	Lactobacillus acidophilus; Bifidobacteria bifidum (bifidus); vitamins B1, B2, B3, B6, B12, K; biotin, inositol	Short-term depletion effects are minimal
	Calcium	Heart/blood pressure irregularities, osteoporosis, tooth decay
	Magnesium	Asthma, cardiovascular problems, cramps, osteoporosis, PMS

DRUG	NUTRIENT DEPLETIONS	POTENTIAL HEALTH PROBLEMS
General antibiotics (continued)	Iron	Anemia, brittle nails, fatigue, hair loss, weakness
Co-trimoxazole	Lactobacillus acidophilus; Bifidobacteria bifidum (bifidus); folic acid	Short-term depletion effects are minimal
Tetracvclines, sulfonamides	Lactobacillus acidophilus; Bifidobacteria bifidum (bifidus); vitamins B1, B2, B3, B6, B12, K; biotin, inositol	Short-term depletion effects are minimal
Neomycin	Beta carotene; Vitamin A, B12	Short-term depletion effects are minimal
Estrogen and hormone replacement therapies		
Estrogen derivatives and selective estrogen receptor modulators	Magnesium	Asthma, cardiovascular problems, cramps, osteoporosis, PMS
	Vitamin B6	Depression, increased cardiovascular disease risk, sleep disturbances
	Zinc	Loss of sense of smell and taste, lower immunity, slow wound healing

Detoxification Nutrients

FUNCTION IN DETOXIFICATION	NUTRIENTS USED
	Vitamin B2 (Riboflavin)
	Vitamin B3 (Niacin)
	Vitamin B6 (Pyridoxine)
	Vitamin B12
Phase 1	Folic Acid
	Glutathione
	Branched-chain Amino Acids
	Flavonoids
	Phospholipids
	Glycine
Phase 2	Taurine
	Glutamine
	Cysteine and N-Acetylcysteine
	Methionine

FOOD SOURCES

Mushrooms, raw almonds, broccoli, spinach, organic chicken, asparagus, wild salmon

Organic chicken, organic turkey, wild salmon, halibut, tuna, lentils, lima beans, asparagus, crimini mushrooms

Wild salmon, organic chicken, spinach, avocado, organic turkey, collard greens, brown rice, green peas

Wild salmon, organic chicken, organic turkey

Lentils, chickpeas, asparagus, spinach, broccoli, lima beans, beets, romaine lettuce

Broccoli, brussel sprouts, cabbage, cauliflower, peaches, watermelon, cinnamon, cardamon, curcumin, avocado

Whey protein

Onion, lettuce, basil, cranberry, garlic, cabbage, kale, brussels sprouts, kohirabi, spinach, asparagus, fennel, soy, scarlet runner bean, lima bean, kidney bean, garden pea, adzuki bean, dill, tea, basil, thyme, cayenne, coriander, peppermint, chamomile, anise

Cabbage, cauliflower, flaxseed

Seaweed, spirulina, sesame seeds, pumpkin seeds, almonds, sunflower seeds, cod, salmon, tuna, turkey, chicken, fenugreek, mustard seed

Cold water fish such as salmon and cod

Cabbage and beets, beans, nuts, fish

Poultry, red peppers, garlic, onions, broccoli, brussel sprouts, oats, wheat germ

Bass trout, cod, beans, garlic, lentils, onions, seeds

Detoxification Nutrients (continued)

FUNCTION IN DETOXIFICATION	NUTRIENTS USED
	Coenzyme Q10
	Thiols
	Silymarin (Milk Thistle)
	Bioflavonoids
	Vitamin A (Carotenes)
	Vitamin C (Ascorbic Acid)
Antioxidant Protective Nutrients and Plant Derivatives	Vitamin E (Tocopherols)
	Selenium
	Copper
	Zinc
	Molybdenum
	Manganese
	Pycnogenol
	Carnosol
Antimicrobials	Allicin
	Phenolic Constituents (carvacrol, thymol)
	Lauric Acid

FOOD SOURCES

Wild fish, lamb, spinach, broccoli, peanuts, wheat germ and whole grains

Garlic, onions, cruciferous vegetables

Silymarin plant

Grapes, berries

Spinach, sweet potatoes, yams, carrots, cod liver oil, butter nut squash, canteloupe, watercress, goji berries

Sweet red pepper, brussel sprouts, cooked broccoli, cooked collard greens, canteloupe, cooked cabbage, tomato, acerola cherries

Cold pressed, extra virgin olive oil; raw almonds; spinach; carrots; avocado; butter; all dark green leafy vegetables

Raw Brazil nuts, wild salmon, brown rice, organic chicken organic beef, organic butter

Raw cashews, raw sunflower seeds, raw hazelnuts, raw almonds organic peanut butter, mushrooms, lentils, whole oats

Lima beans, organic/wild turkey, split peas, chick peas, raw cashews, raw pecans, raw almonds, green peas, ginger root

Beans lentils, peas, whole grains, raw nuts

Pineapple, raw pecans, raw almonds, brown rice, pinto beans, lima beans, navy beans, spinach, sweet potatoes, organic butter fat

Peels, skins, or seeds of grapes, blueberries, cherries, plums

Rosemary

Garlic

Oregano oil

Coconut

CLEAN RESOURCES

TAKING CLEAN FURTHER

Personal Consultations

To consult with Dr. Junger in New York, please contact the Eleven Eleven Wellness Center. If you suspect you are a candidate for the Spent program, arrange to meet with my colleague Dr. Frank Lipman. For consultations in California, please contact the Akasha Wellness Center in Los Angeles. The Akasha team and I work together bi-coastally.

Retreats

If Clean has inspired you to visit a retreat center for a more total-immersion detoxification program, there are several places in the United States that are great for a first or repeat experience. We Care spa in California is world-famous, and deservedly so. Susana Belen, its founder and owner and one of my teachers, has designed a very safe and effective program. Dr. Gabriel Cousens has a center, the Tree of Life, in Arizona, where fasting detox programs are conducted under his supervision. Optimum Health Institute in San Diego,

Hippocrates in Florida, and Sanoviv in Mexico all have different angles on the subject but are all very good.

Web Sites

For further information, the following Web sites are excellent resources:

www.cleanprogram.com. The Clean program online. This Web site will help you navigate your cleanse day by day by providing tips, articles, and links, and you can also order the Clean Kit here. It will also let you document your progress and join a large community of other people doing Clean. There is power in numbers; when you can share your experience and hear what others are doing, the whole process of change can be made even more meaningful.

www.cancerdecisions.com. The best resource I have found for those outside the medical profession are the Moss Reports, exhaustively compiled reports on the latest treatments for and research on every kind of cancer, from the latest in Western medicine to experimental therapies and Eastern modalities. They can be ordered from this site.

www.debraslist.com. There are many sources of information out there about detoxing your home. This is an excellent place to start; you will find many links to other sites and information on research.

Acknowledgments

Thank you . . .

Tierney, for Grace, for your love, and for being a living example of forgiveness and generosity.

My meditation teacher, for resetting my compass and protecting me on my journey.

Muki and Alberto, my parents, for giving me life and an amazing family.

Anabella, my sister, a force without limits, always there for me, even when she was the one in desperate need herself.

Albert Bitton and Hugo Cory, for being my anchors to the present.

Richard Baskin, for his mentoring friendship.

Dr. Frank Lipman, for opening a world of possibilities and the doors to his home and practice. Janice, for her amazing home-cooked soup delivery, thank you.

Fernando Sulichin, my teacher of reinvention.

Amely Greeven, for helping me put my ideas into English.

Claudia Riemer Boutote and Gideon Weil, for your belief, support, and expert guidance.

James Mathers, my esoteric brother and muse.

Dr. Rony Shimony, for proving that even hard-core Western medicine can have magical, way-above-statistical results, when prescribed with a fully open and giving heart.

My earth family, Emilee Barnouin, Michael Barnouin and Walker Blake, Gabriel Raij, Ari Dunski, Vicky and Steven Mendal, Stephanie Junger, Andrea Junger, Doron Junger, Janos Junger, Sybilla Sorondo, Dr. Itzhak and Ziva Kronzon, Dr. Roberto Canessa, Timothy Martin, Jose Luis Longinotti, Dr. Victor Atallah, Tania Landau, Cucu and Andres Levin, Tommie Wright, Myriam and Miguel Baikovicius and all their kids, Andrew Keegan, Jill Pettijohn, Ole, Spoon, Pablo Jourdan, Tenzin Bob Thurman and Nena, Dr. Omar and Reina Burschtin, Dr. Jeffrey James, Raven, Eric Cahan, Jaime Cuevas, Xavier Longueras, Joad Puttermilech, Lilakoi Moon, Andrew Calder, Dr. Steven Gundry, Dr. Voletti, Elena Brower, Skip and Edie Bronson, William Wendling, Gabrielle Roth, Annette Frehling, Donna Karan, Jacqueline and Ted Miller, Yvonne Lasher, Judi Werthein, Brad Listermann, Rachel Goldstein, Herbert Donner, Irene Valenti, Dra Maria Noel Tarabal, Michael Dahan, Gil Barretto, Dra Isabel Llovet, Jack

Curley, Susana Belen, Susie Lombardi, Chabela Lobo, Steven Shailer, Gwyneth Paltrow, the Deambrossi family, Alejandro Curcio, Marcelo Angres, Chicho, Miguel Sirgado, Cindy Palusami, Catherine Parrish, Dr. Steve Sharon, Dr. William and Fran Cole, Jason Harler, Dr. Steven Levine, Dr. Phillip Frankel, Dr. Henry Bellaci, Rafael and Tatiana Bellavita, Martin Fontaina, Dalia Cohn, Lau Pielaat and his boys, Marco Perego, Dhrumil Purohit, Vicky, Anne, Vannessa, and Jessica (my bosses at Eleven Eleven Wellness Center), Prema Dubroff, Miguel Gil, Baretta, Daisy Duck McCrackin, Nicholas Wolfson, Scott Schwenk, Peter Evans, Dr. Edison DeMello, Dr. William So, Timothy Gold, Mary Jenkins, Pali, Natashakti, Chris, Jo, Malaya, Nurse D., Dr. Woodson Merrell, Eric Wilcox, Aryan Morgan, Jako Benmaor.

Last but not least, all my patients, for trusting me, and for providing me with an opportunity to fulfill my passion, to be of service in their journey of healing and transformation.

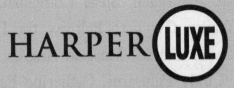
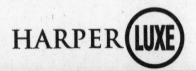